Renal Diet Cookbook for Beginners

160+ Wholesome, Low-Sodium, Low-Potassium, Low-Phosphorus Recipes to Eat Healthy and Avoid Dialysis.
Healthy, Easy and Delicious Recipes!

Sarah Stone

Disclaimer

The content of this book has been checked and compiled with great care. For the completeness, correctness and topicality of the contents however no guarantee or guarantee can be taken over. The content of this book represents the personal experience and opinion of the author and is for entertainment purposes only. The content should not be confused with medical help.

There will be no legal responsibility or liability for damages resulting from counterproductive exercise or errors by the reader. No guarantee can be given for success. The author therefore assumes no responsibility for the non-achievement of the goals described in the bo

Breakfast Recipes

1 Amazing Watermelon-Raspberry Smoothie

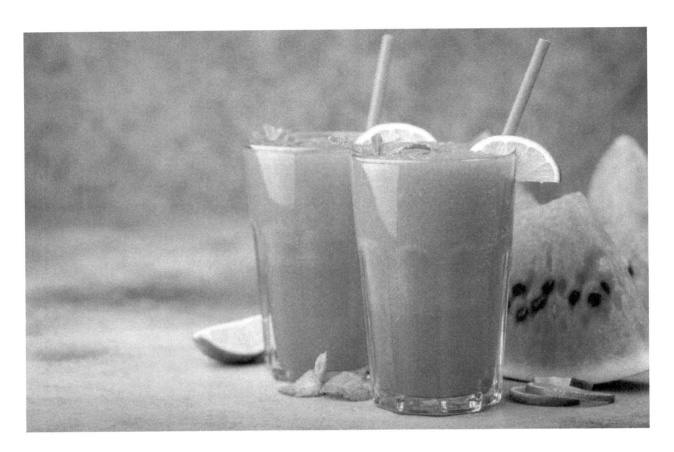

Preparation Time: 30 minutes

Cooking Time: 40 minutes

Servings: 3

Nutritional Content Per Serving:

- Calories: 50
- Fat: 2g
- Carbohydrates: 14g
- Phosphorus: 64mg
- Potassium: 72mg

- Sodium: 37mg
- Protein: 1g

Ingredients:

- Half mug fresh raspberries
- one mug of chopped watermelon
- one mug ice

Instructions:

- In a blender, combine the cabbage and pump for two minutes or until finely chopped. Pulse for about a minute or until the watermelon and raspberries are well mixed.
- Blend in the ice until the smoothie is extremely thick and smooth. Fill two glasses with the mixture and serve.

2   Delicious Apple-Chai Smoothie

Preparation Time: 20 Minutes

Cooking Time: 40 Minutes

Servings: 4

Nutritional Content Per Serving:

- Calories: 88
- Fat: 1g
- Carbohydrates: 19g
- Phosphorus: 74mg
- Potassium: 92mg
- Sodium: 47mg
- Protein: 1g

Ingredients:

- one apple, peeled, cored, and chopped
- one mug not sweetened rice milk
- one chai tea bag
- two mugs ice

Instructions:

- Heat the rice milk in a medium saucepan over low heat for about five minutes or until steaming. Remove the milk from the heat and steep the tea bag.
- Enable 30 minutes for the milk to cool in the refrigerator with the tea bag, remove the tea bag, and squeeze gently to release all flavors. In a blender, combine the milk, apple, and ice and blend until smooth.

3 Tasty Cinnamon-Nutmeg Muffins

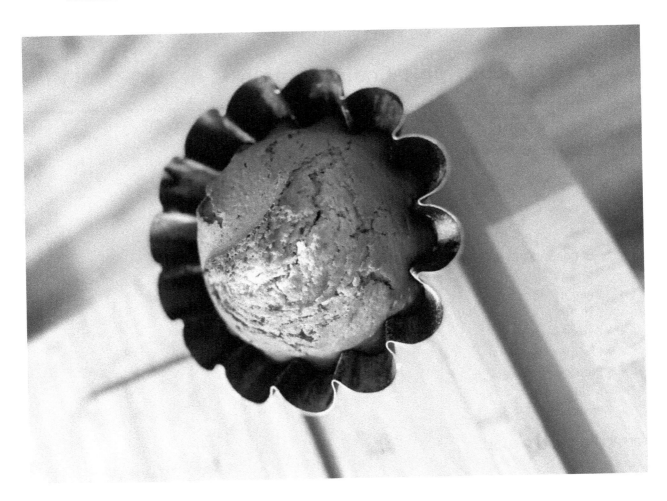

Preparation Time: 40 minutes

Cooking Time: 1 hour

Servings: 6

Nutritional Content Per Serving:

- Calories: 78
- Fat: 1g
- Carbohydrates: 29g
- Phosphorus: 54mg
- Potassium: 52mg
- Sodium: 37mg
- Protein: 2g

Ingredients:

- one tbsp. Ener-G baking soda substitute
- one tsp. ground cinnamon
- Half tsp. ground nutmeg
- Pinch ground ginger
- two mugs, not sweetened rice milk
- one tbsp. apple cider vinegar
- three Half mugs all-purpose flour
- one mug granulated sugar
- Half mug canola oil
- two tbsp. pure vanilla extract
- 2Half mugs fresh blueberries

Instructions:

- Warm up the oven to 375-degree Fahrenheit. Line the mugs of a muffin pan with paper liners; set aside. In a small dish, stir together the rice milk and vinegar; put aside for 10 minutes. In a big dish, stir along with the flour, sugar, baking soda substitute, cinnamon, nutmeg, and ginger until well mixed.
- Add the oil and vanilla to the milk mixture and stir to mix. Add the milk mixture to the dry ingredients and stir until just combined. Fold within the blueberries. Spoon the muffin batter evenly into the mugs. Bake the muffins for 25 to thirty minutes or until golden and a toothpick inserted in the middle of a muffin comes out clean. Allow the muffins to chill for 15 minutes before serving.

4 Simple Fruit and Cheese Breakfast Wrap

Preparation Time: 20 minutes

Cooking Time: 50 minutes

Servings: 3

Nutritional Content Per Serving:

- Calories: 68
- Fat: 1g
- Carbohydrates: 39g
- Phosphorus: 54mg
- Potassium: 42mg
- Sodium: 17mg
- Protein: 3g

Ingredients:

- one apple, peeled, cored, and diced thin
- one tbsp. honey
- two (six-inch) flour tortillas
- two tbsp. plain cream cheddar cheese

Instructions:

- Lay both tortillas on a clean work surface and spread one tbsp. Of cream cheddar cheese onto every tortilla, leaving about half in. around the perimeters. Arrange the apple slices on the cream cheddar cheese, simply off the tortilla's center on the facet closest to you, leaving about 1Half inches on each facet and two inches on the underside.
- Spray the apples lightly with honey. Fold the tortillas' left and right edges into the middle, laying the sting over the apples. Taking the tortilla edge closest to you, fold it over the fruit and the facet items. Roll the tortilla away from you, creating a cozy wrap. Repeat with the second tortilla.

5 Strawberry–Cream Cheese French Toast

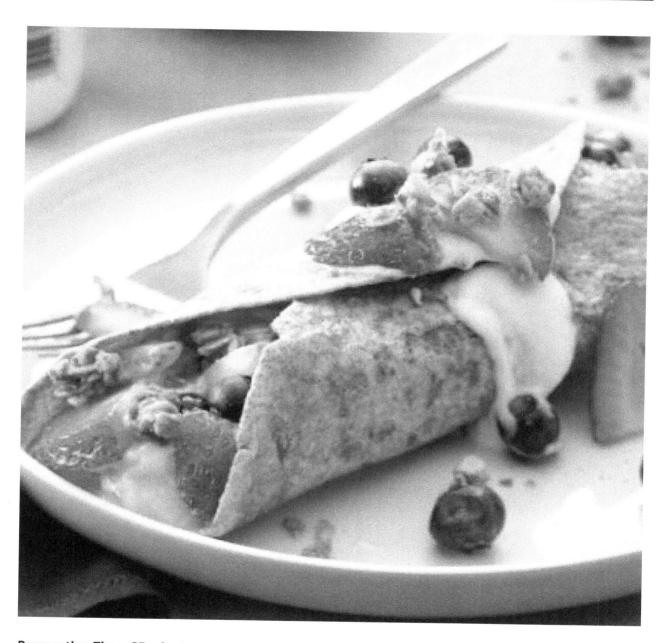

Preparation Time: 25 minutes

Cooking Time: 45 minutes

Servings: 5

Nutritional Content Per Serving:

- Calories: 68
- Fat: 1g
- Carbohydrates: 11g
- Phosphorus: 24mg
- Potassium: 42mg
- Sodium: 27mg
- Protein: 1g

Ingredients:

- two eggs, beaten
- Half mug, not sweetened rice milk
- one tsp. pure vanilla extract
- one tbsp. granulated sugar
- Cooking spray for greasing the baking dish
- Half mug plain cream cheddar cheese
- four tbsp. strawberry jam
- eight slices thick white bread
- one-fourth tsp. ground cinnamon

Instructions:

- Heat the oven to 350-degree Fahrenheit. Spray an eight-by-eight-in. baking dish with cooking spray; set aside. In a little dish, stir along with the cream cheddar cheese and jam until well blended. Spread 3 tbsp. The cream cheddar cheese mixture onto four slices of bread and top with the remaining four slices to create sandwiches. In a moderate dish, stir together the eggs, milk, and vanilla till swish.
- Dip the sandwiches into the egg mixture and lay them in the baking dish. Pour any remaining egg mixture over the sandwiches and sprinkle them evenly with sugar and cinnamon. Cowl the dish with foil and refrigerate overnight. Bake the French toast, covered, for one hour. Separate the foil and bake for five minutes additional or until the French toast is golden. Serve heat.

6 Delicious Vegetable Omelet

Preparation Time: 20 minutes

Cooking Time: 40 minutes

Servings: 3

Nutritional Content Per Serving:

- Calories: 38
- Fat: 2g
- Carbohydrates: 29g
- Phosphorus: 44mg
- Potassium: 62mg
- Sodium: 37mg
- Protein: 1g

Ingredients:

- Olive oil spray for greasing the skillet
- Half mug chopped and boiled red bell pepper
- one-fourth mug chopped scallion, both green and white parts
- four egg whites
- one egg
- two tbsp. chopped fresh parsley
- two tbsp. water
- Freshly ground black pepper

Instructions:

- In a small dish, stir together the egg whites, egg, parsley, and water until well blended; put aside. Generously spray a big nonstick skillet with olive oil spray, and place it over moderate-high heat. Fry the peppers and scallion for regarding 3 minutes or until softened. Pour the egg mixture into the skillet over the vegetables and cook, swirling the skillet, for regarding 2 minutes or until the perimeters of the egg start to the line.
- Raise the set edges and tilt the pan so that the uncooked egg can flow beneath the cooked egg. Continue lifting and cooking the egg for concerning four minutes or until the omelet is ready. Loosen the omelet with a spatula and fold it in. Cut the folded omelet into three parts and transfer the omelets to serving plates. Season with black pepper and serve.

7 Fresh Herbs with Cheesy Scrambled Eggs

Preparation Time: 15 minutes

Cooking Time: 40 minutes

Servings: 4

Nutritional Content Per Serving:

- Calories: 88
- Fat: 1g
- Carbohydrates: 19g

- Phosphorus: 74mg
- Potassium: 92mg
- Sodium: 47mg
- Protein: 1g

Ingredients:

- one tbsp. finely chopped scallion, green part only
- one tbsp. chopped fresh tarragon
- two tbsp. unsalted butter
- three eggs, at room temperature
- two egg whites, at room temperature
- Half mug cream cheddar cheese, at room temperature
- one-fourth mug not sweetened rice milk
- Freshly ground black pepper

Instructions:

- Stir together the eggs, egg whites, cream cheddar cheese, rice milk, scallions, and tarragon in a medium mixing bowl until well combined and smooth.
- Melt the butter in a broad skillet over medium-high heat, stirring to evenly cover the skillet. Prepare, constantly stirring, for about five minutes, or until the eggs are thick and the curds are creamy. Season with salt and pepper.

8 Amazing Egg and Veggie Muffins

Preparation Time: 30 minutes

Cooking Time: 1hour

Servings: 5

Nutritional Content Per Serving:

- Calories: 68
- Fat: 2g
- Carbohydrates: 29g
- Phosphorus: 64mg
- Potassium: 72mg
- Sodium: 37mg
- Protein: 2g

Ingredients:

- Half red bell pepper, finely chopped
- one tbsp. chopped fresh parsley
- Pinch red pepper flakes
- Cooking spray for greasing the muffin pans
- four eggs
- two tbsp. not sweetened rice milk
- Half sweet onion, finely chopped
- Pinch freshly ground black pepper

Instructions:

- Preheat the oven to 350 degrees Fahrenheit (180 degrees Celsius). Set aside four muffin pans that have been sprayed with cooking spray.
- Mix the eggs, milk, onion, red pepper, parsley, red pepper flakes, and black pepper in a large mixing bowl. Fill the muffin tins halfway with the egg mixture. Preheat the oven to 350°F and bake the muffins for 18 to 20 minutes, or until golden and puffed. Serve cold or warm.

9   Tasty Dilly Scrambled Eggs

Preparation Time: 25 minutes

Cooking Time: 50 minutes

Servings: 4

Nutritional Content Per Serving:

- Calories: 78
- Fat: 1g
- Carbohydrates: 29g
- Phosphorus: 64mg
- Potassium: 82mg
- Sodium: 37mg
- Protein: 2g

Ingredients:

- one tsp. dried dill weed
- two big eggs
- one/eight tsp. black pepper
- one tbsp. crumbled goat cheddar cheese

Instructions:

- In a dish, whisk the eggs and pour them into a nonstick skillet over medium heat. Toss eggs with black pepper and dill weed.
- Prepare until the eggs have been scrambled. Until eating, sprinkle with crumbled goat cheddar cheese.

10 Fat Free Great Way to Start Your Day Bagel

Preparation Time: 10 minutes

Cooking Time: 20 minutes

Servings: 4

Nutritional Content Per Serving:

- Calories: 58
- Fat: 2g
- Carbohydrates: 59g
- Phosphorus: 44mg
- Potassium: 62mg
- Sodium: 26mg
- Protein: 1.5g

Ingredients:

- two tomato slices, One-Fourth" thick
- two red onion slices
- one bagel, two-ounce size
- two tbsp. cream cheddar cheese
- one tsp. low-sodium lemon pepper seasoning

Instructions:

- Toast the bagel slices until golden brown. Spread cream cheddar cheese on both halves of the bagel.
- Sprinkle with lemon pepper and finish with onion and tomato slices.

11 Apple Oatmeal Custard

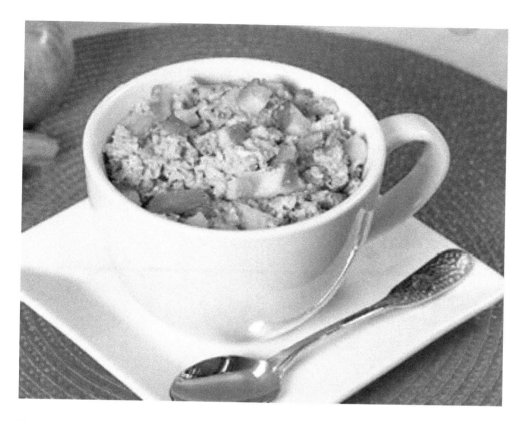

Preparation Time: 10 minutes

Cooking Time: 20 minutes

Servings: 2

Nutritional Content Per Serving:

- Calories: 84
- Fat: 1.2g
- Carbohydrates: 14g
- Phosphorus: 73mg
- Potassium: 52mg
- Sodium: 34mg
- Protein: 2g

Ingredients:

- One-Fourth tsp. cinnamon

- Half moderate apple
- one/three mug quick-cooking oatmeal
- one big egg
- Half mug almond milk

Instructions:

- Half an apple, cored and finely chopped in a large mug, combine the oats, egg, and almond milk. With a fork, thoroughly combine the ingredients. Toss in the apple and cinnamon. Stir once more until it is well combined.
- Prepare for two minutes on high in the microwave. Using a fork, fluff the mixture. If necessary, cook for another 30 to 60 seconds. If you want a thinner cereal, add a little more milk or water.

12 Breakfast Pancakes

Preparation Time: 20 minutes

Cooking Time: 40 minutes

Servings: 4

Nutritional Content Per Serving:

- Calories: 76
- Fat: 1.5 g
- Carbohydrates: 29g
- Phosphorus: 34mg
- Potassium: 56mg
- Sodium: 23mg
- Protein: 1g

Ingredients:

- two tsp. (nine gram) sodium-free baking powder, one egg
- one mug (235 milliliters) milk
- one-fourth mugs (145 gram), all-purpose flour
- two tbsp. (26 gram) sugar
- one tbsp. (15 milliliters) vegetable oil

Instructions:

- Mix the dry ingredients in a mixing bowl. Mix the egg, milk, and oil in a mixing bowl. Both of the ingredients should be added to the flour mixture at the same time. Stir until well combined but somewhat lumpy.
- For each pancake, pour about one-fourth mug of batter onto a hot, greased griddle. Prepare until the bottom is browned (when bubbles form and then break). Prepare until cooked on the other side.

13 Breakfast Waffles

Preparation Time: 30 minutes

Cooking Time: 1 hour

Servings: 5

Nutritional Content Per Serving:

- Calories: 45
- Fat: 2g
- Carbohydrates: 46g
- Phosphorus: 56mg
- Potassium: 76mg
- Sodium: 43mg
- Protein: 2g

Ingredients:

- one egg
- third-fourth mug (175 milliliters) skim milk
- one tbsp. (14 gram) unsalted butter
- one mug (110 gram) all-purpose flour
- one tsp. sodium-free baking powder
- one tsp. sugar

Instructions:

- Mix egg, milk, and melted butter. Add to dry ingredients, mixing until just blended. Do not overbeat. Bake according to waffle iron directions.

14 Amazing Apple Pancakes

Preparation Time: 20 minutes

Cooking Time: 40 minutes

Servings: 4

Nutritional Content Per Serving:

- Calories: 56
- Fat: 2g
- Carbohydrates: 19g
- Phosphorus: 65mg
- Potassium: 67mg
- Sodium: 31mg
- Protein: 1g

Ingredients:

- two eggs
- one mug (235 milliliters), skim milk
- one mug (245 gram), applesauce
- one-Half mugs (165 gram), all-purpose flour
- two tbsp. (26 gram) sugar
- one tbsp. (14 gram) sodium-free baking powder
- one-fourth tsp. ground nutmeg
- two tbsp. (28 gram) unsalted butter, melted

Instructions:

- In a large mixing bowl, combine the dry ingredients. Combine the eggs, milk, applesauce, and butter in a mixing bowl. Stir in the wet ingredients until just combined, still lumpy.
- Heat the grill and pour about a quarter of a mug (60 milliliters) of batter per pancake. Prepare until the bubbles have exploded. Prepare until golden brown on the other hand.

15 Tasty Baked French Toast

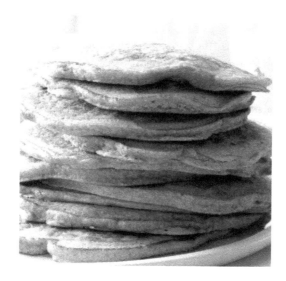

Preparation Time: 15 minutes

Cooking Time: 20 minutes

Servings: 4

Nutritional Content Per Serving:

- Calories: 78
- Fat: 1g
- Carbohydrates: 49g
- Phosphorus: 54mg
- Potassium: 32mg
- Sodium: 34mg
- Protein: 1g

Ingredients:

- Half mug (60 gram) all-purpose flour
- six tbsp. (90 gram) brown sugar
- Half tsp. the ground cinnamon, packed
- one-fourth mug (55 gram) unsalted butter
- six slices low sodium bread
- three eggs
- three tbsp. (39 gram) sugar

- one tsp. vanilla extract
- two one-fourth mugs (535 milliliters) skim milk
- one mug (145 gram) blueberries, fresh or frozen

Instructions:

- Cut bread into one-in. (2. 5 cm)-thick slices and place during a greased nine × 13-in. (23 × thirty-three-cm) baking dish. In a very moderate dish, gently beat eggs, sugar, and vanilla. Stir within the milk until well blended. Pour over bread, turning pieces to coat well.
- Cover and refrigerate overnight. Warm-up oven to 375-degree Fahrenheit (190 degree Celsius, gas mark 5). During a tiny dish, mix the flour, brown sugar, and cinnamon. Cut in butter until the mixture resembles coarse crumbs. Flip bread over in baking dish. Scatter blueberries over bread. Sprinkle evenly with crumb mixture. Bake for concerning 40 minutes till golden brown.

16 Banana Fritters

Preparation Time: 10 minutes

Cooking Time: 20 minutes

Servings: 4

Nutritional Content Per Serving:

- Calories: 65
- Fat: 1g
- Carbohydrates: 34g
- Phosphorus: 43mg
- Potassium: 45mg
- Sodium: 23mg
- Protein: 1g

Ingredients:

- one egg
- one tbsp. (15 milliliters) canola oil
- one mug (225 gram) banana, chopped
- one mug (110 gram) all-purpose flour
- one tbsp. (15 gram) sugar
- one tbsp. (14 gram) sodium-free baking powder
- Half mug (120 milliliters) skim milk
- Half tsp. ground nutmeg

Instructions:

- Combine the flour, sugar, and baking powder in a mixing dish. Combine the milk, egg, and oil in a mixing bowl. Combine the banana and nutmeg in a mixing bowl.
- Stir only until the dry ingredients are moistened. Drop tablespoonfuls of dough into the hot oil. Fry each side for two to three minutes until golden brown.

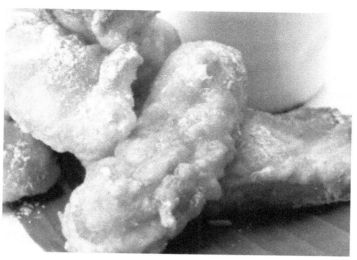

17 Cinnamon Pull-Apart Loaf

Preparation Time: 20 minutes

Cooking Time: 40 minutes

Servings: 4

Nutritional Content Per Serving:

- Calories: 65
- Fat: 1g
- Carbohydrates: 19g
- Phosphorus: 65mg
- Potassium: 92mg
- Sodium: 34mg
- Protein: 1g

Ingredients:

- two-third mug (157 milliliters)
- skim milk two tbsp. (28 gram) unsalted butter
- one tsp. vanilla extract
- four tbsp. (60 gram) sugar divided
- one Hafts. ground cinnamon

- three Half mugs (385 gram) Buttermilk Baking Mix
- one egg
- Half mug (50 gram) powdered sugar
- two tbsp. (30 milliliters) water

Instructions:

- Combine two tbsp. Sugar and also the cinnamon. Place during a resealable plastic bag. Spray a loaf pan with nonstick vegetable oil spray. Stir along with the baking mix, milk, remaining sugar, butter, vanilla, and egg till it forms a ball. Pinch off one Half-inch (four-cm) items.
- Shake in the cinnamon-sugar mixture till coated and then place within the pan. Bake at 375-degree Fahrenheit (190 degree Celsius, gas mark 5) for 25 to thirty minutes or until golden brown. Let stand in pan for 10 minutes before removing. Combine powdered sugar and water and drizzle over high.

18 Delicious Cinnamon Rolls

Preparation Time: 30 minutes

Cooking Time: 1 hour

Servings: 4

Nutritional Content Per Serving:

- Calories: 88
- Fat: 1g
- Carbohydrates: 19g
- Phosphorus: 74mg
- Potassium: 92mg
- Sodium: 47mg
- Protein: 1g

Ingredients:

- one-fourth mug (50 gram) sugar
- 3tsp. (12 gram) yeast
- one-third mug (67 gram) sugar
- two tsp. (five-gram) ground cinnamon
- one mug (235 milliliters) water
- two tbsp. (28 milliliters) vegetable oil
- one egg
- three mugs (330 gram) bread flour
- two tbsp. (28 gram) unsalted butter softened

Instructions:

- Place dough ingredients in the bread machine in the order specified by the manufacturer. A process on the dough cycle. Separate dough and press out to a rectangle on a gently floured board. Mix along with cinnamon and sugar.
- Spread dough with softened butter, then sprinkle with cinnamon-sugar mixture. Roll up tightly, starting on the nine-inch (23-cm) facet. Slice into nine slices. Place cut facet down in an exceedingly greased nine × 9-inch baking pan. Cover and let rise till doubled, 30 to forty-five minutes. Bake at 375-degree Fahrenheit (one hundred ninety-degree Celsius, gas mark five) till golden, 25 to thirty minutes.

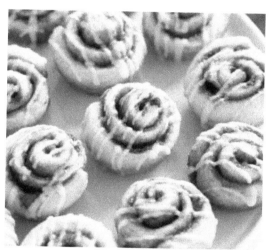

19 Low Carb Honey-Topped Coffee Cake

Preparation Time: 20 minutes

Cooking Time: 40 minutes

Servings: 3

Nutritional Content Per Serving:

- Calories: 76
- Fat: 2g
- Carbohydrates: 23g
- Phosphorus: 45mg
- Potassium: 76mg
- Sodium: 33mg
- Protein: 1g

Ingredients:

- Half tsp. mace
- one can (eight third-fourth oz., or 255 gram) pineapple,
- one-fourth mug (60 milliliters) vegetable oil
- one-Half mugs (165 gram) all-purpose flour
- Half mug (100 gram) sugar
- two tsp. (nine gram) sodium-free baking powder
- one-third mug (115 gram) honey Half mug (57 gram) granola
- one-fourth mug (18 gram) coconut

Instructions:

- Combine the dry ingredients in a mixing dish. Drain the pineapple and preserve the syrup. If required, add water to the syrup to make half a mug.
- Combine the syrup, egg, and oil in a mixing bowl. Stir in the flour mixture until it is fully smooth. Fill a round baking pan with the batter that has been coated with nonstick vegetable oil spray. Combine the honey, pineapple, granola, and coconut in a bowl. Cover the batter with the sauce.

20 Low Fat Apple Strata

Preparation Time: 20 minutes

Cooking Time: 30 minutes

Servings: 4

Nutritional Content Per Serving:

- Calories: 88
- Fat: 1g
- Carbohydrates: 19g
- Phosphorus: 34mg
- Potassium: 32mg
- Sodium: 33mg
- Protein: 1g

Ingredients:

- three oz. (85 gram) Swiss cheddar cheese,
- three mugs, low sodium bread, cubed
- one can (15 oz., or 455 gram) apples
- four eggs
- one-fourth mug (60 milliliters) skim milk

Instructions:

- Cube bread and place in a very 9-in.-square (twenty-three-cm-sq.) pan sprayed with nonstick vegetable oil spray. Spoon apples over bread. Sprinkle with cheddar cheese. Mix eggs and milk and pour over bread, apples, and cheddar cheese.
- Cowl with plastic wrap and refrigerate overnight. Warm-up oven to 350-degree Fahrenheit (one hundred eighty degree Celsius, gas mark four). Bake uncovered for 40 to forty-five minutes or until high is lightly browned, and the center is ready.

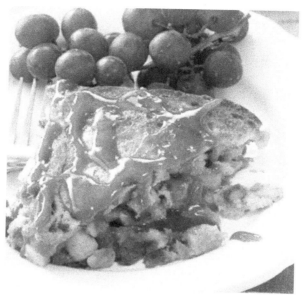

21 Low Sodium Sausage Gravy

Preparation Time: 30 minutes

Cooking Time: 1 hour

Servings: 3

Nutritional Content Per Serving:

- Calories: 77
- Fat: 1g
- Carbohydrates: 55g
- Phosphorus: 67mg
- Potassium: 76mg
- Sodium: 35mg
- Protein: 1g

Ingredients:

- Half lb. (225 gram) Sausage

- one mug (235 milliliters) skim milk
- one-fourth tsp. black pepper
- three tbsp. (24 gram) all-purpose flour

Instructions:

- Separate sausage with a slotted spoon; set aside. Separate all but two tbsp. (28 milliliters) of grease from the skillet. Over moderate heat, stir three tbsp. (24 gram) of flour into the grease. Stir constantly until browned, about five minutes.
- Stirring constantly, pour in the milk. Season with pepper. Continue stirring until the gravy is thick. Add sausage back into the gravy. Serve over split biscuits, grits, or mashed potatoes, or pour into a dish or gravy boat and serve on the side.

22 Special Breakfast Burritos

Preparation Time: 20 minutes

Cooking Time: 45 minutes

Servings: 5

Nutritional Content Per Serving:

- Calories: 67
- Fat: 1g
- Carbohydrates: 35g
- Phosphorus: 33mg
- Potassium: 24mg
- Sodium: 11mg
- Protein: 1g

Ingredients:

- six flour tortillas
- one mug (110 gram) Swiss cheddar
- one-fourth mug (45 gram) tomato, chopped
- two tbsp. (30 gram) sour cream
- one moderate potato
- Half lb. (225 gram) Sausage one tiny onion, chopped
- one tsp. Chili powder
- one-fourth tsp. cayenne pepper
- two eggs

Instructions:

- Prepare potato in boiling water for 35 minutes until tender. When cool, peel and cut into cubes. Brown sausage in frying pan and add onion, chili powder, and cayenne pepper. Prepare for ten minutes. Drain and discard fat.
- Add cubed, cooked potato. Beat eggs and add to the pan. Stir until eggs are set. Spoon mixture into center of warmed tortilla, high with shredded cheddar cheese, and roll up the tortilla to enclose mixture. For an authentic Mexican bit, serve topped with tomato, sour cream, and salsa.

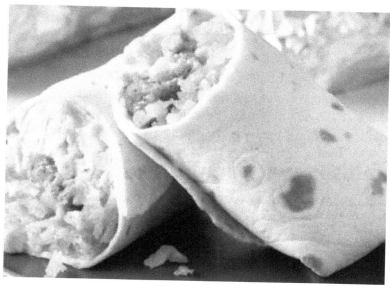

23 Quick Soft Granola Bars

Preparation Time: 10 minutes

Cooking Time: 25 minutes

Servings: 4

Nutritional Content Per Serving:

- Calories: 66
- Fat: 1g
- Carbohydrates: 12g
- Phosphorus: 14mg
- Potassium: 13mg
- Sodium: 10mg
- Protein: 1g

Ingredients:

- one-fourth mug (60 milliliters) corn syrup
- one-fourth mug (85 gram) honey

- Half mug (82. five-gram) raisins
- Half mug (35 gram) sweetened coconut
- three mugs (240 gram) quick-cooking oats
- Half mug (115 gram) brown sugar
- one-fourth mug (28 gram) wheat germ
- Half mug (112 gram) unsalted butter

Instructions:

- Combine the oats, sugar, and wheat germ in a mixing bowl. Add the butter and proceed to cut until the mixture is crumbly. Combine the corn syrup and honey in a mixing bowl.
- Combine the raisins and coconut in a bowl. In a greased 9-inch (23-cm) square pan, press the dough. Bake for 20 to 25 minutes at 350 degrees Fahrenheit (180 degrees Celsius, gas mark four). Enable to cool for 10 minutes before cutting into bars.

24 Proteins Power Bars

Preparation Time: 20 minutes

Cooking Time: 30 minutes

Servings: 4

Nutritional Content Per Serving:

- Calories: 90
- Fat: 1g
- Carbohydrates: 34g
- Phosphorus: 33mg
- Potassium: 23mg
- Sodium: 25mg
- Protein: 1g

Ingredients:

- one-fourth mug (60 gram) applesauce
- one-fourth mug (85 gram) honey
- three tbsp. (45 gram) brown sugar
- two tbsp. (30 milliliters) vegetable oil
- one-fourth mug (56 gram) sunflower seeds, unsalted
- one mug (80 gram) quick-cooking oats
- Half mug (75 gram) whole wheat flour
- Half mug (57 gram) Grape-Nuts cereal, or other nugget-type cereal
- Half tsp. ground cinnamon

- one egg
- one-fourth mug (35 gram) walnuts, chopped
- seven oz. (198 gram) dried fruit

Instructions:

- Warm-up oven to 325-degree Fahrenheit (a hundred and seventy degree Celsius, gas mark three). Line a 9-inch (twenty-three-cm) square baking pan with aluminum foil. Spray the foil with cooking spray. In a big dish, stir along with the oats, flour, cereal, and cinnamon.
- Add the egg, applesauce, honey, brown sugar, and oil. Mix well. Stir within the sunflower seeds, walnuts, and dried fruit. Spread mixture evenly in the ready pan. Bake for 30 minutes, or till firm and gently browned around the edges. Let cool. Use the foil to elevate from the pan. Cut into bars and store within the refrigerator.

25 Simple Breakfast Mix

Preparation Time: 20 minutes

Cooking Time: 20 minutes

Servings: 4

Nutritional Content Per Serving:

- Calories: 78
- Fat: 1g
- Carbohydrates: 24g
- Phosphorus: 21mg
- Potassium: 22mg
- Sodium: 11mg
- Protein: 1g

Ingredients:

- three tbsp. (60 gram) honey,
- three tbsp. (45 milliliters) corn syrup
- one tbsp. (14 gram) unsalted butter
- one tsp. ground cinnamon
- two mugs (200 gram) bite-size frosted shredded wheat cereal
- two mugs (200 gram) Kellogg's Crackling' Oat Bran
- peanuts
- Half mug (82. five-gram) raisins
- two mugs unsalted pretzels
- one-fourth tsp. ground nutmeg

Instructions:

- In a large mixing bowl, combine cereal, almonds, raisins, and pretzels. Combine the sugar, corn syrup, butter, and spices in a mixing bowl. Microwave until the water is boiling. Pour over the cereal mixture and stir to combine.
- Place in a pan that hasn't been greased. Preheat oven to 325°F (170°C, gas mark 3) and bake for 20 minutes, stirring after 10 minutes. Place on waxed paper to cool. Separate and allow to cool. Keep the jar airtight.

26 Milky Breakfast Biscuits

Preparation Time: 20 minutes

Cooking Time: 12 minutes

Servings: 5

Nutritional Content Per Serving:

- Calories: 89
- Fat: 1g
- Carbohydrates: 22g
- Phosphorus: 33mg
- Potassium: 42mg
- Sodium: 13mg
- Protein: 1g

Ingredients:

- Half tsp. cream of tartar
- Half mug (112 gram) unsalted butter
- two mugs (220 gram) all-purpose flour
- 4tsp. (18 gram) sodium-free baking powder two tsp. (eight gram) sugar
- two-third mug (157 milliliters) skim milk

Instructions:

- Combine the first four ingredients in a mixing bowl. Using a pastry cutter, cut in the butter until the mixture resembles coarse crumbs. Pour in the milk. Stir until it is evenly distributed. Knead a few times on a floured surface.
- Press to a thickness of half an inch (one-fourth of a centimeter). Cut out two half-inch (six.25-cm) biscuits with two half-inch (six.25-cm) biscuit cutters. Transfer to a baking sheet that hasn't been greased. Bake for 10 to 12 minutes at 450 degrees Fahrenheit (230 degrees Celsius, gas mark 8).

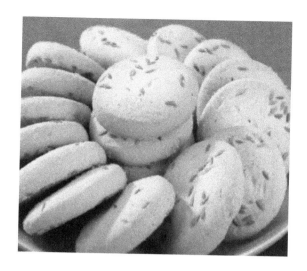

27 Amazing Restaurant-Style Biscuits

Preparation Time: 20 minutes

Cooking Time: 25 minutes

Servings: 3

Nutritional Content Per Serving:

- Calories: 85
- Fat: 1g
- Carbohydrates: 21g
- Phosphorus: 21mg
- Potassium: 15mg
- Sodium: 17mg
- Protein: 1g

Ingredients:

- two mugs (220 gram) Buttermilk Baking Mix
- two oz. (60 gram) sour cream
- Half mug (120 milliliters) club soda

Instructions:

- Combine the baking mix, sour cream, and club soda in a mixing bowl. Lightly knead the dough on a lightly floured surface. Roll or pat to a thickness of half an inch (one-fourth of a centimeter). Using a biscuit cutter or a sharp knife, break the dough into six biscuits.
- Spray an eight-inch (20-cm) baking dish with nonstick vegetable oil spray and place biscuits in it. Pour melted butter over the top. Preheat oven to 375 degrees Fahrenheit.

28 Simple Cheddar Biscuits

Preparation Time: 20 minutes

Cooking Time: 12 minutes

Servings: 4

Nutritional Content Per Serving:

- Calories: 88
- Fat: 1g
- Carbohydrates: 19g
- Phosphorus: 74mg
- Potassium: 92mg
- Sodium: 47mg
- Protein: 1g

Ingredients:

- two-third mug (157 milliliters) skim milk Half mug (58 gram)
- mug (55 gram) unsalted butter, melted
- one-fourth tsp. garlic powder
- two mugs (220 gram) all-purpose flour
- one tbsp. (14 gram) sodium-free baking powder
- four tbsp. (55 gram) unsalted butter
- Half tsp. dried parsley

Instructions:

- Combine the flour and baking powder in a mixing dish. Using a pastry cutter, cut in the butter until the mixture resembles coarse crumbs.
- Mix in the milk and cheddar cheese until it is well mixed. Bake for 10 to 12 minutes at 400 degrees Fahrenheit (200 degrees Celsius, gas mark 6) on a greased baking dish. Pour hot biscuits with melted butter, garlic powder, and parsley. Squares should be cut out.

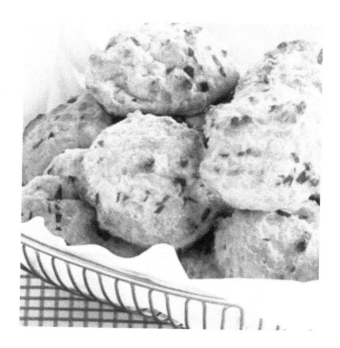

29 Low Fat Sweet Potato Biscuits

Preparation Time: 30 minutes

Cooking Time: 15 minutes

Servings: 3

Nutritional Content Per Serving:

- Calories: 78
- Fat: 1g
- Carbohydrates: 20g
- Phosphorus: 70mg
- Potassium: 15mg
- Sodium: 11mg
- Protein: 1g

Ingredients:

- two tbsp. (28 gram) unsalted butter
- third-fourth mug (169 gram) sweet potatoes, mashed
- one-fourth mug (60 milliliters) skim milk one mug (110 gram) all-purpose flour
- 3tsp. (14 gram) sodium-free baking powder two tsp. (eight gram) sugar

Instructions:

- Warm up the oven to four hundred-degree Fahrenheit (two hundred degree Celsius, gas mark six). In a moderate dish, stir together the flour, baking powder, and sugar. Cut within the butter till pieces of butter are pea-size or smaller.
- Mix within the sweet potatoes and enough of the milk to make a soft dough. Turn dough out onto a floured surface, and roll or pat out to Half-in. (one one-fourth-cm) thickness. Cut into circles using a biscuit cutter or a drinking glass. Place biscuits one inch (2. Five cm) apart onto a greased baking sheet. Bake for 12 to fifteen minutes in the preheated oven, or till golden brown.

30 Low Sodium Cornbread

Preparation Time: 15 minutes

Cooking Time: 25 minutes

Servings: 2

Nutritional Content Per Serving:

- Calories: 77
- Fat: 1g
- Carbohydrates: 12g
- Phosphorus: 15mg
- Potassium: 67mg
- Sodium: 37mg
- Protein: 1g

Ingredients:

- one tbsp. (14 gram) sodium-free baking powder
- one mug (140 gram) cornmeal
- one mug (110 gram) all-purpose flour
- one-fourth mug (50 gram) sugar
- one-fourth mug (55 gram) unsalted butter
- one mug (235 milliliters) skim milk
- one egg

Instructions:

- Combine the first four ingredients in a mixing bowl. Using a pastry cutter, cut in the butter until the mixture resembles crumbs.
- Stir together the milk and egg, then add to the dry ingredients, stirring only until combined. Bake for 20 to 25 minutes at 425 degrees Fahrenheit (220 degrees Celsius, gas mark 7) in a nine-inch (23-cm) square pan sprayed with nonstick vegetable oil spray.

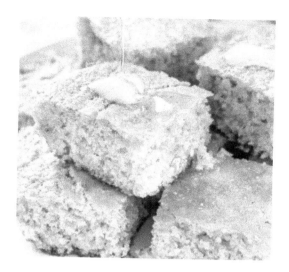

31 Delicious Creamed Celery and Peas

Preparation Time: 20 minutes

Cooking Time: 10 minutes

Servings: 3

Nutritional Content Per Serving:

- Calories: 78
- Fat: 1g
- Carbohydrates: 29g
- Phosphorus: 34mg
- Potassium: 12mg
- Sodium: 27mg
- Protein: 1g

Ingredients:

- Half mug (115 gram) sour cream
- Half tsp. dried rosemary
- One-Eighth tsp. garlic powder
- one-third mug (80 milliliters) water
- two mugs (200 gram) celery, diced
- 10 oz. (280 gram) no-salt-added frozen peas
- one-fourth mug (31 gram) slivered almonds

Instructions:

- Bring the water to a boil in a saucepan. Cook for eight minutes after adding the celery. Return to a boil with the peas.
- Cook for another three minutes, covered. Drain the water. Combine the sour cream and spices in a mixing bowl and blend well. In a serving bowl, arrange the vegetables. Serve with a dollop of sour cream on top. Almonds, if desired.

32 Delightful Fresh Veggie Medley

Preparation Time: 20 minutes

Cooking Time: 10 minutes

Servings: 3

Nutritional Content Per Serving:

- Calories: 89
- Fat: 1g
- Carbohydrates: 17g
- Phosphorus: 73mg
- Potassium: 45mg
- Sodium: 11mg
- Protein: 1g

Ingredients:

- one zucchini, cubed
- one-fourth tsp. garlic powder
- Half lb. (225 gram) green beans
- four tomatoes, chopped
- one tsp. dried basil

Instructions:

- Wash, trim and cook beans until almost tender. Drain. Return to pan with other mentioned ingredients and cook to desired doneness.

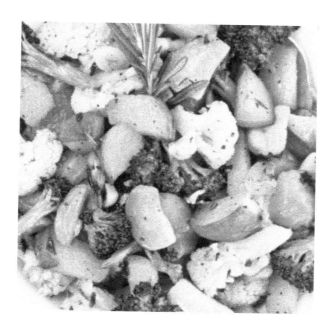

33 Simple Green Bean Casserole

Preparation Time: 20 minutes

Cooking Time: 35 minutes

Servings: 3

Nutritional Content Per Serving:

- Calories: 56
- Fat: 1g
- Carbohydrates: 19g
- Phosphorus: 14mg
- Potassium: 12mg
- Sodium: 17mg
- Protein: 1g

Ingredients:

- One-eight tsp. pepper
- 10 oz. (280 gram) Condensed Cream of Mushroom Soup
- 18 oz. (504 gram) frozen green beans
- Half mug (80 gram) onion, chopped
- two tbsp. (30 milliliters) vegetable oil
- one-fourth mug (60 milliliters) skim milk
- Half mug (65 gram) French-fried onions

Instructions:

- Fry onion in oil until tender. Mix all ingredients except French-fried onions in a one Half-quart (one Half-L) casserole. Bake at 350-degree Fahrenheit (180 degree Celsius, gas mark four) for 30 minutes. Sprinkle French-fried onions on top. Bake for five minutes longer.

34 Grilled Vegetable Packs

Preparation Time: 20 minutes

Cooking Time: 40 minutes

Servings: 3

Nutritional Content Per Serving:

- Calories: 79
- Fat: 1g
- Carbohydrates: 19g
- Phosphorus: 56mg
- Potassium: 45mg
- Sodium: 34mg
- Protein: 1g

Ingredients:

- one-fourth tsp. black pepper
- one-fourth tsp. garlic powder
- two mugs, zucchini, diced
- two onions, peeled and diced
- two mugs (260 gram) carrot, diced

Instructions:

- Divide the vegetables into four large aluminum foil squares. Using a teaspoon of water, wet each packet. Season with salt, pepper, and garlic.
- Fold each packet in half and firmly close it. Grill for about 40 minutes over moderate coals, turning periodically until vegetables are tender.

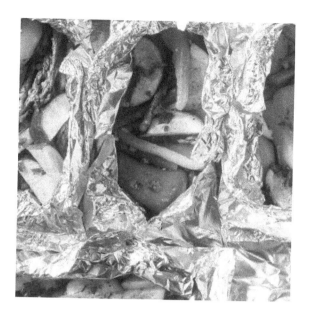

35 Low carb Marinated Carrots

Preparation Time: 20 minutes

Cooking Time: 35 minutes

Servings: 4

Nutritional Content Per Serving:

- Calories: 78
- Fat: 1g
- Carbohydrates: 29g
- Phosphorus: 44mg
- Potassium: 22mg
- Sodium: 24mg
- Protein: 1g

Ingredients:

- third-fourth mug (175 milliliters) water
- one tbsp. (11 gram) mustard seed
- two mugs (260 gram), carrots
- third-fourth mug (150 gram) sugar
- third-fourth mug (175 milliliters) vinegar
- one stick cinnamon
- three whole cloves

Instructions:

- Carrots should be cooked for five minutes. Drain and slice into three-inch (7.5-cm) sticks. Get the remaining ingredients to a boil. Cook for 10 minutes on low heat.
- Overnight in the refrigerator, pour over carrots, cover, and refrigerate. Drain, then serve.

36 Curried Fresh Vegetables

Preparation Time: 20 minutes

Cooking Time: 30 minutes

Servings: 3

Nutritional Content Per Serving:

- Calories: 77
- Fat: 1g
- Carbohydrates: 29g
- Phosphorus: 54mg
- Potassium: 42mg
- Sodium: 37mg
- Protein: 1g

Ingredients:

- Half mug (60 gram) green bell pepper, coarsely chopped
- one-fourth tsp. garlic powder
- one tbsp. (six. Three gram) curry powder
- three mugs (540 gram) tomatoes, chopped
- Half mug (80 gram) onion, coarsely chopped
- one mug zucchini, cubed

Instructions:

- Mix all ingredients in a saucepan. Prepare and stir until vegetables are softened. Serve with mint sauce.

37 Oriental Vegetable Toss

Preparation Time: 10 minutes

Cooking Time: 10 minutes

Servings: 3

Nutritional Content Per Serving:

- Calories: 89
- Fat: 1g
- Carbohydrates: 23g
- Phosphorus: 34mg
- Potassium: 33mg
- Sodium: 22mg
- Protein: 1g

Ingredients:

- four oz. (115 gram) mushrooms, diced
- Half mug (60 gram) red bell pepper, diced
- four oz. (115 gram) mung bean sprouts
- one-fourth mug (60 milliliters) Soy Sauce
- Half lb. (225 gram) lettuce, shredded
- four oz. (115 gram) snow peas
- Half mug (65 gram) carrot, diced
- one mug (70 gram) cabbage, shredded
- two tbsp. (30 milliliters) mirin wine
- Half tsp. ground ginger
- one tbsp. (eight gram) sesame seeds

Instructions:

- Toss salad and mentioned ingredients. Spoon dressing over. Serve with mint sauce.

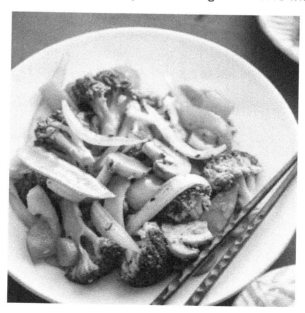

38 Amazing Roasted Beets

Preparation Time: 30 minutes

Cooking Time: 25 minutes

Servings: 3

Nutritional Content Per Serving:

- Calories: 67
- Fat: 1g
- Carbohydrates: 39g
- Phosphorus: 44mg
- Potassium: 22mg
- Sodium: 17mg
- Protein: 1g

Ingredients:

- one tsp. olive oil
- two beets, well-scrubbed but not peeled
- one tsp. dried thyme

Instructions:

- Preheat the oven to 450 degrees Fahrenheit (230 degrees Celsius) (230 degree Celsius, gas mark eight). Remove the beets' tops and root ends before slicing them as thinly as possible (aim for one-eighth-inch [0.32 cm]).
- Toss the beet slices with the olive oil in a medium bowl, then finish with a sprinkling of thyme. Roast beets in a single layer on one or two baking sheets for 20 to 25 minutes in a preheated oven.

39 Roasted Mexican Vegetables

Preparation Time: 10 minutes

Cooking Time: 20 minutes

Servings: 3

Nutritional Content Per Serving:

- Calories: 88
- Fat: 1g

- Carbohydrates: 29g
- Phosphorus: 34mg
- Potassium: 32mg
- Sodium: 37mg
- Protein: 1g

Ingredients:

- Half onion, diced into wedges
- Half green bell pepper, cut into one-inch (two. Five-cm) pieces
- Half mug (90 gram) plum tomatoes split in half
- two tbsp. (28 milliliters) olive oil
- , one clove garlic, minced
- Half tsp. dried basil
- Half tsp. dried oregano
- one mug zucchini, cut in one-inch (two. Five-cm) slices
- four oz. (115 gram) mushrooms, cut in half
- Nonstick vegetable oil spray

Instructions:

- In a resealable plastic container, combine the oil, garlic, basil, and oregano. Shake to uniformly cover the vegetables. Using cooking spray, coat a nine 13-inch (23-33-cm) roasting pan.
- In the pan, arrange the vegetables in a single layer. Roast for 20 minutes at 400 degrees Fahrenheit (200 degrees Celsius, gas mark 6) until crisp fried.

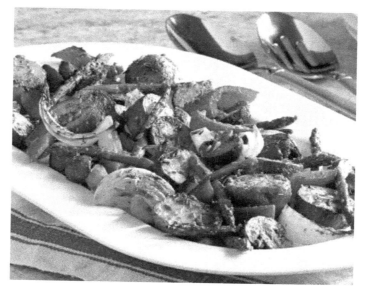

40 Delicious Veggie Hash

Preparation Time: 20 minutes

Cooking Time: 30 minutes

Servings: 4

Nutritional Content Per Serving:

- Calories: 77
- Fat: 1g
- Carbohydrates: 23g
- Phosphorus: 22mg
- Potassium: 27mg
- Sodium: 13mg
- Protein: 1g

Ingredients:

- one-fourth mug zucchini, shredded
- two tbsp. (28 milliliters) olive oil
- two potatoes, shredded
- Half mug (80 gram) onion, shredded
- one-fourth mug (30 gram) red bell pepper, shredded
- one-fourth mug (30 gram) green bell pepper, shredded
- one-third mug (60 gram) tomatoes, finely chopped

Instructions:

- Except for the tomatoes, combine all of the vegetables in a large mixing bowl. In a large skillet, heat the oil. Spread out the vegetables in an even layer.
- Cook until the edges are finely browned. Turnover and cover with chopped tomatoes. Cook, wrap until the vegetables are tender. To serve, cut into wedges.

41 Low Sodium Spanish Green Beans

Preparation Time: 10 minutes

Cooking Time: 10 minutes

Servings: 3

Nutritional Content Per Serving:

- Calories: 69
- Fat: 1g
- Carbohydrates: 15g
- Phosphorus: 16mg

- Potassium: 17mg
- Sodium: 18mg
- Protein: 1g

Ingredients:

- one mug (180 gram) tomatoes, chopped
- Half tsp. dried basil
- Half tsp. dried rosemary
- Half lb. (225 gram) green beans
- one-fourth mug (40 gram) onion, chopped
- one-fourth mug (30 gram) green bell pepper, chopped
- one tbsp. (15 milliliters) olive oil

Instructions:

- Prepare beans in boiling water until tender. Drain and set aside. Fry onion and pepper in oil until soft. Add tomatoes and spices. Stir in beans. Warm-up through.

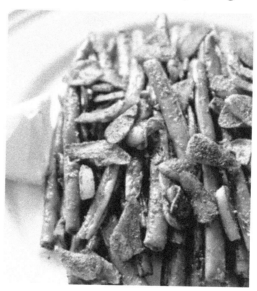

42 Sweet and Sour Red Cabbage

Preparation Time: 30 minutes

Cooking Time: 7 hours

Servings: 4

Nutritional Content Per Serving:

- Calories: 77
- Fat: 1g
- Carbohydrates: 29g
- Phosphorus: 34mg
- Potassium: 52mg
- Sodium: 37mg
- Protein: 1g

Ingredients:

- Half mug (115 gram) brown sugar
- Half mug (120 milliliters) cider vinegar
- four mugs (280 gram), red cabbage, shredded
- one onion, chopped
- one apple, peeled and chopped

Instructions:

- Put vegetables in a slow cooker. Mix sugar and vinegar, pour over vegetables and stir to mix. Prepare on low for seven to eight hours.

43 Tasty Grilled Onions

Preparation Time: 30 minutes

Cooking Time: 40 minutes

Servings: 3

Nutritional Content Per Serving:

- Calories: 88
- Fat: 1g
- Carbohydrates: 19g
- Phosphorus: 74mg
- Potassium: 92mg
- Sodium: 47mg
- Protein: 1g

Ingredients:

- two tsp. (10 milliliters) sodium-free beef bouillon
- two onions
- two tbsp. (28 gram) unsalted butter
- Half tsp. garlic powder

Instructions:

- Onions should be peeled. Create a tiny hole in the middle of each onion by slicing a small section off one end. Fill one tsp. bouillon, one tbsp. (14 gramme) butter, and one-fourth tsp. garlic powder into the center of each onion.
- Wrap the onion in aluminum foil and replace the top. Close the grill after placing the onions on a preheated moderate grill. Cook for one hour or until the meat is tender.

44 Baked Beans

Preparation Time: 30 minutes

Cooking Time: 40 minutes

Servings: 4

Nutritional Content Per Serving:

- Calories: 90
- Fat: 1g
- Carbohydrates: 29g
- Phosphorus: 34mg
- Potassium: 42mg
- Sodium: 46mg
- Protein: 1g

Ingredients:

- two tbsp. (40 gram) molasses
- two tbsp. (30 gram) brown sugar
- one, Hafts. dry mustard
- Half lb. (225 gram) navy beans
- four mugs (940 milliliters) water
- one mug (240 gram) Chili Sauce
- third-fourth mug (120 gram) onion, chopped
- one-fourth tsp. garlic powder
- one mug (235 milliliters) water

Instructions:

- Place beans in water in a big saucepan. Bring to a boil and cook for one minute. Separate from the heat and let stand for one hour.
- Return to heat and simmer until almost done about one hour. Drain. Mix with remaining ingredients. Place in a one Half-quart (one Half-L) baking dish. Cover and bake for four hours. Add water if needed during cooking.

45 Curried Chickpeas

Preparation Time: 20 minutes

Cooking Time: 15 minutes

Servings: 4

Nutritional Content Per Serving:

- Calories: 88
- Fat: 1g
- Carbohydrates: 19g
- Phosphorus: 34mg
- Potassium: 92mg
- Sodium: 36mg
- Protein: 1g

Ingredients:

- four mugs (400 gram) chickpeas, cooked
- Half tsp. turmeric
- Half tsp. cumin
- one tbsp. (11 gram) mustard seed
- one tbsp. (15 milliliters) olive oil
- Dash red pepper flakes
- Half mug (80 gram) shallots, minced
- one-fourth tsp. ground ginger
- one-fourth mug (15 gram) fresh cilantro

Instructions:

- Mustard seeds should be fried in oil in a large saucepan before they start to pop. Sauté the shallots and red pepper flakes until the shallots are tender.
- Add the chickpeas, turmeric, cumin, and ginger, as well as enough water to keep the mixture from sticking. Simmer for 15 minutes before serving, garnished with cilantro.

46 Baked Sweet Potatoes

Preparation Time: 30 minutes

Cooking Time: 45 minutes

Servings: 4

Nutritional Content Per Serving:

- Calories: 86
- Fat: 1g
- Carbohydrates: 19g
- Phosphorus: 54mg
- Potassium: 32mg
- Sodium: 27mg
- Protein: 1g

Ingredients:

- one-fourth mug (60 gram) brown sugar
- four sweet potatoes
- one tsp. ground cinnamon

Instructions:

- Scrub potatoes and score the skin with a knife to allow the steam to escape. Bake at 375-degree Fahrenheit (190 degree Celsius, gas mark five) until done, about 45 minutes. Sprinkle with brown sugar and cinnamon.

47 Delightful Caribbean Sweet Potatoes

Preparation Time: 20 minutes

Cooking Time: 35 minutes

Servings: 4

Nutritional Content Per Serving:

- Calories: 76
- Fat: 1g
- Carbohydrates: 19g
- Phosphorus: 44mg
- Potassium: 46mg
- Sodium: 25mg
- Protein: 1g

Ingredients:

- one-fourth mug (60 gram) brown sugar
- one-fourth mug (60 milliliters) orange juice
- two tsp. (10 milliliters) lime juice

- two sweet potatoes, peeled and cubed
- one tsp. vegetable oil
- one-fourth mug (30 gram) red bell pepper, chopped
- one-fourth mug (40 gram) onion, chopped
- one Hafts. Jerk Seasoning

Instructions:

- In a pot of boiling water, cook sweet potatoes until they are just tender. Drain thoroughly. In a large skillet, heat the oil. In a large mixing bowl, add the sweet potatoes, bell pepper, and onion.
- In a small bowl, combine the sugar, juices, and seasoning. Return the juice mixture to the pan with the vegetables and cook over medium heat until the liquid has reduced to a syrupy consistency.

48 Western Omelet in a Mug

Preparation Time: 30 minutes

Cooking Time: 40 minutes

Servings: 4

Nutritional Content Per Serving:

- Calories: 77
- Fat: 1g
- Carbohydrates: 29g
- Phosphorus: 34mg
- Potassium: 32mg
- Sodium: 22mg
- Protein: 1g

Ingredients:

- one tbsp. (nine gram) chopped green bell pepper
- Half mug (125 gram) egg substitute, or two eggs, beaten
- two tbsp. (14 gram) shredded Swiss cheddar cheese
- two tbsp. (20 gram) chopped onion

Instructions:

- Spray a microwave-safe mug with nonstick cooking spray, then add all of the ingredients and mix well. Microwave for one minute on high, uncovered; stir.
- Cook for another one to one and a half minutes, or until the eggs are fully set.

49 Low Fat Devilish Mexican Eggs

Preparation Time: 20 minutes

Cooking Time: 35 minutes

Servings: 4

Nutritional Content Per Serving:

- Calories: 90
- Fat: 1g
- Carbohydrates: 39g
- Phosphorus: 44mg
- Potassium: 52mg
- Sodium: 17mg
- Protein: 1g

Ingredients:

- One-Fourth tsp. freshly ground black pepper
- One-Fourth mug (28 gram) shredded Swiss cheddar cheese
- one mug (260 gram) Low-Sodium Salsa two eggs

Instructions:

- Simmer the salsa in a tiny skillet over moderate heat. Crash in the eggs, cover, and heat until the whites set; top with the pepper and cheddar cheese.

50 Herb Enhanced Eggs

Preparation Time: 15 minutes

Cooking Time: 30 minutes

Servings: 3

Nutritional Content Per Serving:

- Calories: 67
- Fat: 1g
- Carbohydrates: 11g
- Phosphorus: 13mg
- Potassium: 15mg

- Sodium: 17mg
- Protein: 1g

Ingredients:

- one tbsp. (four-gram) minced fresh parsley
- one tbsp. (five-gram) grated Parmesan cheddar cheese
- four eggs
- One-Fourth tsp. minced garlic
- One-Fourth tsp. minced fresh thyme
- One-Fourth tsp. minced fresh rosemary
- two tbsp. (30 milliliters) cream
- one tbsp. (14 gram) unsalted butter
- One-Fourth tsp. freshly ground black pepper

Instructions:

- Warm up the broiler and place the oven rack six inches (fifteen cm) below the heat supply. Mix the garlic, thyme, rosemary, parsley, and Parmesan and put aside. Carefully crack two eggs into each of 2 small bowls without breaking the yolks.
- Place two individual gratin dishes on a baking sheet. Place one tbsp. (15 milliliters) of cream and Half tbsp. of butter in every dish and broil for concerning three minutes, till hot and bubbly. Quickly but fastidiously, pour the eggs into every gratin dish, sprinkle evenly with the herb mixture, and then sprinkle with the pepper. Broil for five to 6 minutes longer until the whites of the eggs are almost cooked. The eggs can continue to cook once you're taking them out of the oven. Allow setting for sixty seconds before serving.

51 Asian Frittata

Preparation Time: 30 minutes

Cooking Time: 45 minutes

Servings: 3

Nutritional Content Per Serving:

- Calories: 67
- Fat: 1g
- Carbohydrates: 23g
- Phosphorus: 22mg
- Potassium: 21mg
- Sodium: 24mg
- Protein: 1g

Ingredients:

- Half mug (125 gram) egg substitute, or two eggs, beaten
- two tsp. chopped fresh herbs, or Half tsp. dried
- one/eight tsp. freshly ground black pepper
- one mug (160 gram) chopped onion
- One-Fourth mug (60 milliliters) water
- one tsp. oil
- two tbsp. (31 gram) ricotta cheddar cheese

Instructions:

- Bring the onion and water to a boil in a very small nonstick skillet over moderate-high heat. Cover and cook till the onion are slightly softened for two minutes. Uncover and continue cooking till the water has evaporated, one to two minutes longer. Spray in the oil and stir to coat. Continue cooking, stirring typically, until the onion starts to brown, one to two minutes a lot of.
- Pour within the egg, reduce the warmth to moderate-low, and continue cooking, constantly stirring, till the egg is starting to line, concerning 20 seconds. Continue cooking, lifting the perimeters; thus, the uncooked egg will flow beneath, till mostly set, regarding thirty seconds more. Cut back the warmth to low. Sprinkle the herbs and pepper over the frittata. Spoon the ricotta on top. Lift an edge of the frittata and drizzle regarding one tbsp. (fifteen milliliters) water underneath it.
- Cowl and cook till the egg are completely set, and also the cheddar cheese is hot, for 2 minutes. Slide the frittata out of the pan using a spatula and serve.

52 Cheesy Hash Brown Skillet Breakfast

Preparation Time: 30 minutes

Cooking Time: 40 minutes

Servings: 3

Nutritional Content Per Serving:

- Calories: 65
- Fat: 1g
- Carbohydrates: 13g
- Phosphorus: 18mg
- Potassium: 22mg
- Sodium: 21mg
- Protein: 1g

Ingredients:

- Half mug (125 gram) egg substitute, or two eggs
- One-Fourth tsp. freshly ground black pepper
- one tbsp. (15 milliliters) olive oil
- one mug (115 gram) frozen hash browns
- four oz. (115 gram) frozen spinach, thawed and drained
- One-Fourth mug (28 gram) shredded Swiss cheddar cheese

Instructions:

- In a small nonstick skillet, heat the oil over medium heat. In a pan, layer the hash browns and spinach. Pour the egg over the top, then season with pepper and cheddar cheese.
- Cover and cook for four to seven minutes, or until the hash browns are beginning to brown on the bottom, the egg is set, and the cheddar cheese is melted.

53 Open-Faced Mexican Breakfast Sandwich

Preparation Time: 30 minutes

Cooking Time: 20 minutes

Servings: 3

Nutritional Content Per Serving:

- Calories: 77
- Fat: 1g
- Carbohydrates: 29g
- Phosphorus: 64mg
- Potassium: 42mg
- Sodium: 37mg
- Protein: 1g

Ingredients:

- Bread toasted two tbsp. (33 gram) Low-Sodium Salsa
- One-Fourth mug (63 gram) Refried Beans two Slices Low-Sodium Whole Wheat
- two tbsp. (14 gram) shredded Swiss cheddar cheese

Instructions:

- Place the refried beans on the toast. Top with the salsa, then the cheddar cheese. Microwave on high until the cheddar cheese is melted and the beans are hot for about 45 seconds.

54 Breakfast Tomato-Egg Scramble

Preparation Time: 20 minutes

Cooking Time: 15 minutes

Servings: 3

Nutritional Content Per Serving:

- Calories: 88
- Fat: 1g
- Carbohydrates: 19g
- Phosphorus: 74mg
- Potassium: 92mg
- Sodium: 47mg
- Protein: 1g

Ingredients:

- one mug (180 gram) chopped tomatoes
- one tsp. chopped fresh basil
- one tbsp. (14 gram) unsalted butter
- two mugs (500 gram) egg substitute, or eight eggs, beaten
- One-Fourth tsp. freshly ground black pepper

Instructions:

- In a large skillet, melt the butter over medium heat. Pour in the beaten eggs and scramble until the eggs are almost done, stirring vigorously with a wooden spoon.
- Cook, constantly stirring, for one minute, until the tomatoes are heated through and beginning to soften. Season with salt and pepper to taste, and serve right away.

55 Veggie and Egg Scramble for One

Preparation Time: 20 minutes

Cooking Time: 15 minutes

Servings: 3

Nutritional Content Per Serving:

- Calories: 76

- Fat: 1g
- Carbohydrates: 29g
- Phosphorus: 34mg
- Potassium: 42mg
- Sodium: 17mg
- Protein: 1g

Ingredients:

- One-Fourth mug (63 gram) egg substitute, or one egg, beaten
- One-Fourth mug (19 gram) diced mushrooms
- Half mug (80 gram) frozen pepper and onion mix
- One-Fourth mug (28 gram) shredded Swiss cheddar cheese

Instructions:

- Cook the mushrooms and frozen vegetables in a small skillet coated with nonstick cooking spray for two to three minutes until cooked through.
- Pour the egg into the skillet and gently stir until it is completely cooked for about 5 minutes. Remove from the heat and cover for two minutes to allow the cheddar cheese to melt.

56 Breakfast Quesadillas

Preparation Time: 20 minutes

Cooking Time: 30 minutes

Servings: 4

Nutritional Content Per Serving:

- Calories: 66
- Fat: 1g
- Carbohydrates: 29g
- Phosphorus: 34mg
- Potassium: 22mg
- Sodium: 16mg
- Protein: 1g

Ingredients:

- One-Fourth mug (65 gram) Low-Sodium Salsa One-Fourth mug (30 gram)
- one mug (250 gram) egg substitute, or four eggs, beaten
- eight corn tortillas

Instructions:

- Coat a skillet with nonstick spray, add the eggs, and scramble over moderate heat, stirring within the salsa and cheddar cheese once they are almost set, for four to 5 minutes. Lightly coat one side of the tortillas with olive oil cooking spray and place four oil facet down on a baking sheet.
- Divide the egg mixture among the tortillas, spreading to a good thickness. Top with the remaining tortillas, oil side up. Grill the quesadillas till heated through and golden brown, about three minutes per facet. Cut into quarters to serve.

57 Farina and Almonds

Preparation Time: 30 minutes

Cooking Time: 20 minutes

Servings: 2

Nutritional Content Per Serving:

- Calories: 57
- Fat: 1g
- Carbohydrates: 22g
- Phosphorus: 43mg
- Potassium: 34mg
- Sodium: 14mg
- Protein: 1g

Ingredients:

- one tbsp. (15 gram) packed brown sugar
- two tbsp. (18 gram) roasted unsalted almonds
- two mugs (470 milliliters) skim milk
- one/three mug farina (40 gram), such as Cream of Wheat (not instant)

Instructions:

- In a small saucepan over high heat, bring the milk to a boil. In a separate bowl, whisk together the flour and the milk.
- Reduce the heat to low and cook, whisking regularly, for two to three minutes, or until the sauce has thickened. Spoon into bowls and uniformly spread the sugar, apricots, and almonds.

58 Quick Peanut Butter and Banana Breakfast

Preparation Time: 20 minutes

Cooking Time: 15 minutes

Servings: 2

Nutritional Content Per Serving:

- Calories: 77
- Fat: 1g
- Carbohydrates: 50g
- Phosphorus: 34mg
- Potassium: 32mg
- Sodium: 17mg
- Protein: 1g

Ingredients:

- one Slice Low-Sodium Whole Wheat Bread, toasted one banana, diced
- two tsp. no-salt-added peanut butter

Instructions:

- Add the peanut butter to the warm toast. Serve with the diced banana. Serve with honey.

59 Crunchy Yogurt Parfaits

Preparation Time: 20 minutes

Cooking Time: 15 minutes

Servings: 3

Nutritional Content Per Serving:

- Calories: 88
- Fat: 1g
- Carbohydrates: 19g
- Phosphorus: 74mg
- Potassium: 92mg
- Sodium: 47mg
- Protein: 1g

Ingredients:

- two mugs (460 gram) low-fat strawberry yoghurt
- Half mug (75 gram) strawberries

- one mug (55 gram) mini shredded wheat cereal, crumbled

Instructions:

- Slice all but two of the strawberries. Place a layer of strawberry slices in each of two parfait glasses. Sprinkle One-Fourth mug cereal over the strawberries.
- Pour about Half a mug (115 gram) yoghurt over the cereal. Make another layer of strawberries, cereal, and yoghurt. Top each with a whole strawberry.

60 Dessert for Breakfast Ambrosia

Preparation Time: 15 minutes

Cooking Time: 20 minutes

Servings: 4

Nutritional Content Per Serving:

- Calories: 66
- Fat: 1g
- Carbohydrates: 10g
- Phosphorus: 56mg
- Potassium: 52mg
- Sodium: 17mg
- Protein: 1g

Ingredients:

- four mugs (600 gram) peeled and cubed apples
- one mug (110 gram) pecans, coarsely chopped
- two oz. (55 gram) shredded coconut
- four mugs (640 gram) cubed cantaloupe
- four mugs (600 gram) orange sections
- four mugs (600 gram) diced bananas
- One-Fourth mug (60 milliliters) orange juice
- one mug (225 gram) low-fat vanilla yoghurt

Instructions:

- In a big dish, arrange layers of cantaloupe, orange sections, bananas, apples, pecans, and coconut. Mix the orange juice and yoghurt and pour-over. Chill before serving.

61 Special Mixed Fruit Smoothie

Preparation Time: 20 minutes

Cooking Time: 15 minutes

Servings: 2

Nutritional Content Per Serving:

- Calories: 75
- Fat: 1g
- Carbohydrates: 29g
- Phosphorus: 56mg
- Potassium: 44mg
- Sodium: 41mg
- Protein: 1g

Ingredients:

- one mug (145 gram) blueberries
- two mugs (300 gram) diced bananas
- two mugs of low-fat peach yoghurt

Instructions:

- Place all the ingredients in a blender and process until smooth. Serve immediately.

62 Baked Apples with Walnuts

Preparation Time: 10 minutes

Cooking Time: 15 minutes

Servings: 2

Nutritional Content Per Serving:

- Calories: 79
- Fat: 1g
- Carbohydrates: 29g
- Phosphorus: 24mg
- Potassium: 22mg
- Sodium: 17mg

- Protein: 1g

Ingredients:

- Half tsp. ground nutmeg
- 6tsp. (30 gram) unsalted butter
- two-third mug (157 milliliters) apple cider
- six apples
- six tbsp. (90 gram) brown sugar
- Half mug (75 gram) unsalted walnuts, chopped
- Half tsp. ground cinnamon

Instructions:

- Fill each apple cavity with one tablespoon (15 gramme) brown sugar, then break walnuts equally between the cavities. Sprinkle the walnuts with cinnamon and nutmeg, and fill each cavity with a teaspoon of butter.
- Place the apples in an ovenproof baking dish and cover them with hot cider or juice. Bake for 50 to 60 minutes at 375 degrees Fahrenheit (190 degrees Celsius, gas mark 5) in a preheated oven.

63 Vegetable Medley

Preparation Time: 10 minutes

Cooking Time: 15 minutes

Servings: 2

Nutritional Content Per Serving:

- Calories: 87
- Fat: 1g
- Carbohydrates: 34g
- Phosphorus: 24mg
- Potassium: 22mg
- Sodium: 17mg
- Protein: 1g

Ingredients:

- Half mug (80 gram) chopped onion
- Half tsp. sugars
- Half tsp. dillweed
- two big Russet potatoes, peeled and chopped
- 12 oz. (336 gram) frozen corn kernels, thawed

- one-Half mugs (270 gram) seeded and chopped tomato
- one mug (130 gram) diced carrot
- one/eight tsp. freshly ground black pepper

Instructions:

- Coat the inside of a three-quart (three-L) slow cooker with cooking spray. Mix all the ingredients in the slow cooker. Cover and cook on low for five to six hours or until the vegetables are tender.

64 Asian Spaghetti Squash

Preparation Time: 14 minutes

Cooking Time: 12 minutes

Servings: 3

Nutritional Content Per Serving:

- Calories: 85
- Fat: 1g
- Carbohydrates: 29g
- Phosphorus: 44mg
- Potassium: 12mg
- Sodium: 17mg
- Protein: 1g

Ingredients:

- one can (14. five oz., or 411 gram) no-salt-added tomatoes
- One-Fourth tsp. freshly ground black pepper
- , one moderate spaghetti squash
- eight oz. (225 gram) mushrooms, diced
- three/four mug (90 gram) shredded mozzarella cheddar cheese

Instructions:

- Coat the within of a four-to 5-quart (four-to five-L) slow cooker with cooking spray. Cut the squash in 0.5 lengthwise and scoop out and discard the seeds. Place the squash, cut aspect up, in the slow cooker. Layer on the mushrooms and tomatoes and sprinkle with the oregano and pepper. Cover and cook on low for 6 to eight hours or until the squash is tender.
- Sprinkle with the cheddar cheese. Cover and cook for fifteen minutes longer or until the cheddar cheese is melted. When the squash is cool enough to handle, separate into strands with two forks.

65 Grilled Corn

Preparation Time: 15 minutes

Cooking Time: 10 minutes

Servings: 3

Nutritional Content Per Serving:

- Calories: 74
- Fat: 1g
- Carbohydrates: 16g
- Phosphorus: 17mg
- Potassium: 21mg
- Sodium: 22mg
- Protein: 1g

Ingredients:

- four ears corn
- Half tsp. black pepper
- one-fourth mug (55 gram) unsalted butter

Instructions:

- Add the butter to the corn and sprinkle with pepper. Covering in heavy-duty aluminum foil and grill until done, about 15 minutes, turning frequently.

Chapter 3: Breakfast Gluten Free

66 Gluten Free Blueberry-Pineapple Smoothie

Preparation Time: 15 minutes

Cooking Time: 10 minutes

Servings: 2

Nutritional Content Per Serving:

- Calories: 65
- Fat: 1g
- Carbohydrates: 29g
- Phosphorus: 44mg
- Potassium: 32mg
- Sodium: 27mg
- Protein: 1g

Ingredients:

- Half mug English cucumber
- Half apple
- one mug of frozen blueberries
- Half mug pineapple chunks
- Half mug waters

Instructions:

- In a blender, combine the blueberries, pineapple, cucumber, apple, and water until smooth and thick. Fill two glasses with the mixture and serve.

67 Fat Free Corn Pudding

Preparation Time: 20 minutes

Cooking Time: 40 minutes

Servings: 4

Nutritional Content Per Serving:

- Calories: 66
- Fat: 1g
- Carbohydrates: 29g
- Phosphorus: 24mg
- Potassium: 22mg
- Sodium: 17mg
- Protein: 1g

Ingredients:

- third-fourth mug not sweetened rice milk, at room temperature
- three tbsp. Unsalted butter melted
- two tbsp. light sour cream
- Unsalted butter, for greasing the baking dish
- two tbsp. all-purpose flour
- Half tsp. Ener-G baking soda substitute
- three eggs
- two tbsp. granulated sugar
- two mugs frozen corn kernels, thawed

Instructions:

- Warm up the oven to 350-degree Fahrenheit. Lightly grease an eight-by-eight-in. Baking dish with butter; put aside. In a small dish, stir together the flour and baking soda substitute; put aside. In a moderate dish, stir together the eggs, rice milk, butter, bitter cream, and sugar. Stir the flour mixture into the egg mixture until sleek.
- Add the corn to the batter and stir until terribly well mixed. Spoon the batter into the baking dish and bake for 40 minutes or till the pudding is about. Let the pudding cool for about fifteen minutes and serve warm.

68 Low Carb Tofu and Egg Stir-Fry

Preparation Time: 20 minutes

Cooking Time: 40 minutes

Servings: 3

Nutritional Content Per Serving:

- Calories: 96
- Fat: 1g
- Carbohydrates: 29g
- Phosphorus: 21mg
- Potassium: 32mg
- Sodium: 33mg
- Protein: 1g

Ingredients:

- Half mug (125 gram) egg substitute, or two eggs
- One-Fourth tsp. freshly ground black pepper to taste
- four oz. (115 gram) firm tofu
- , two tiny red potatoes
- , two tbsp. (30 milliliters) olive oil
- one tsp. chili powder
- two oz. (55 gram) fresh spinach

Instructions:

- Slice the tofu lengthwise into slices regarding half an inch (one. 3 cm) thick and wrap during a paper towel. Add under one thing significant, such as a dish. Chop the potatoes into little items, place in a microwave-safe dish, fill with water, and microwave for 5 minutes. Place the olive oil in an exceedingly wok and heat to terribly hot over high heat. During a tiny dish, beat the eggs, chili powder, and pepper.
- Chop the spinach into little items. Unwrap the tofu and chop it into tiny items. Drain the potatoes and increase the recent wok. Stir once to thoroughly coat in oil and then let brown on every aspect, stirring only often. Add the tofu to the wok. Completely stir the potatoes and tofu together. Reduce the warmth to moderate. Add the eggs and spinach and stir thoroughly. Let cook for another 3 minutes until the eggs are set.

69 Low Sodium Granola and Yogurt Parfait

Preparation Time: 20 minutes

Cooking Time: 30 minutes

Servings: 3

Nutritional Content Per Serving:

- Calories: 88
- Fat: 1g
- Carbohydrates: 19g
- Phosphorus: 74mg

- Potassium: 92mg
- Sodium: 47mg
- Protein: 1g

Ingredients:

- three/four mug (195 gram) low-fat vanilla yoghurt
- Half mug (85 gram) diced strawberries
- two tbsp. (30 gram) granola

Instructions:

- Add Into two parfait glasses or wine glasses, spoon some berries, vanilla yoghurt, and granola. Repeat the layering until all the ingredients are used. Serve immediately.

70 Tasty Cream-Style Corn

Preparation Time: 30 minutes

Cooking Time: 20 minutes

Servings: 3

Nutritional Content Per Serving:

- Calories: 86
- Fat: 1g
- Carbohydrates: 12g
- Phosphorus: 15mg
- Potassium: 32mg
- Sodium: 11mg
- Protein: 1g

Ingredients:

- one-Half mugs (195 gram) frozen corn, cooked, divided
- two tbsp. (26 gram) sugar

Instructions:

- In a blender, combine half a mug (65 grammes) of cooked corn, one-fourth mug (60 milliliters) cooking liquid, and the sugar (adjust to taste).
- Process until the mixture is mostly liquefied. Attach the remaining mug of corn and process for a few seconds at medium speed, only until the kernels are broken up.

71 Gluten Free Breakfast Tacos

Preparation Time: 20 minutes

Cooking Time: 35 minutes

Servings: 3

Nutritional Content Per Serving:

- Calories: 76
- Fat: 1g
- Carbohydrates: 15g
- Phosphorus: 71mg
- Potassium: 43mg
- Sodium: 44mg
- Protein: 1g

Ingredients:

- Swiss cheddar cheese, shredded
- eight taco shells
- four eggs
- one-fourth mug (56 gram)

Instructions:

- When the eggs are almost done, stir in the salsa and cheddar cheese. Divide the mixture into taco shells and position them upright in an eight-inch (20-cm) baking dish.
- Microwave for one minute or heat for five minutes at 350 degrees Fahrenheit (180 degrees Celsius, gas mark four).

72 Fat free Peanut Butter and Honey Crispy Squares

Preparation Time: 35 minutes

Cooking Time: 20 minutes

Servings: 4

Nutritional Content Per Serving:

- Calories: 74
- Fat: 1g

- Carbohydrates: 12g
- Phosphorus: 24mg
- Potassium: 12mg
- Sodium: 17mg
- Protein: 1g

Ingredients:

- two tbsp. (30 gram) firmly packed brown sugar
- three mugs (75 gram) crispy rice cereal
- one/three mug (87 gram) no-salt-added peanut butter
- One-Fourth mug (55 gram) unsalted butter
- One-Fourth mug (80 gram) honey

Instructions:

- Grease an eight-in. (20-cm) sq. pan. During a saucepan, combine the peanut butter, butter, honey, and brown sugar and convey to a boil over moderate-high heat. Reduce the heat to moderate and boil for one minute, stirring constantly.
- Pour over the cereal in a very massive dish. Press firmly into the prepared pan. Cut into sixteen 2-inch (5-cm) squares. Store during a tightly covered container within the refrigerator.

73 Tasty Funnel Cakes

Preparation Time: 30 minutes

Cooking Time: 20 minutes

Servings: 3

Nutritional Content Per Serving:

- Calories: 76
- Fat: 1g
- Carbohydrates: 11g
- Phosphorus: 21mg
- Potassium: 33mg
- Sodium: 22mg
- Protein: 1g

Ingredients:

- two tbsp. (26 gram) sugar
- one tsp. sodium-free baking powder
- one egg

- two-third mug (157 milliliters) skim milk
- one one-fourth mugs (145 gram) all-purpose flour
- one-fourth mug (25 gram) confectioners' sugar

Instructions:

- Beat egg with milk. Blend flour, sugar, and baking powder and gradually add egg mixture, beating until sleek. Heat at least one in. (two. 5 cm) of oil in a skillet or deep fryer to 375-degree Fahrenheit (190 degree Celsius, gas mark five).
- Place thumb over a bottom gap of the funnel. Pour batter in. Separate thumb and drop into hot oil using a circular motion to spiral about four inches (ten cm) in diameter for each cake. Separate when golden brown. Whereas the cake remains warm, sprinkle with confectioners' sugar. Serve heat.

74 Delightful Skillet-Baked Pancake

Preparation Time: 35 minutes

Cooking Time: 20 minutes

Servings: 2

Nutritional Content Per Serving:

- Calories: 68
- Fat: 1g
- Carbohydrates: 21g
- Phosphorus: 22mg
- Potassium: 23mg
- Sodium: 23mg
- Protein: 1g

Ingredients:

- one-fourth tsp. ground cinnamon
- Pinch ground nutmeg
- two eggs
- Half mug not sweetened rice milk
- Half mug all-purpose flour
- Cooking spray for greasing the skillet

Instructions:

- Heat the oven to 450-degree Fahrenheit. In a moderate dish, stir together the eggs and rice milk. Stir in the flour, cinnamon, and nutmeg till blended but still slightly lumpy; however, do not overmix. Spray a 9-inch ovenproof skillet with cooking spray and place the skillet within the preheated oven for five minutes.

- Separate the skillet fastidiously and pour the pancake batter into the skillet. Return the skillet to the oven and bake the pancake for concerning 20 minutes or till it is overpriced and crispy on the edges. Cut the pancake into halves to serve.

75 Cranberry Upside-Down Cake

Preparation Time: 20 minutes

Cooking Time: 35 minutes

Servings: 3

Nutritional Content Per Serving:

- Calories: 76
- Fat: 1g
- Carbohydrates: 34g
- Phosphorus: 42mg
- Potassium: 32mg
- Sodium: 17mg
- Protein: 1g

Ingredients;

- one mug (110 gram) all-purpose flour
- one Hafts. sodium-free baking powder
- Half mug (125 gram) applesauce
- one egg
- two mugs (220 gram) cranberries
- third-fourth mugs (350 gram) sugar, divided
- Half mug (120 milliliters) water
- one-fourth mug (60 milliliters) skim milk
- one-fourth mug (60 milliliters) orange juice
- one tsp. orange peel, grated
- Half tsp. vanilla extract

Instructions:

- Spray bottom and sides of nine-inch (twenty-three-cm) round baking pan with nonstick vegetable oil spray. Combine cranberries, one mug (200 gram) of sugar, and the water in a huge saucepan. Bring to a boil. Reduce heat and simmer till slightly thickened to a syrupy consistency, about ten minutes.

- Pour into a prepared pan. Cool to space temperature. Sift and flour, remaining third-fourth mug (150 gram) sugar, and baking powder in a very massive dish. In another dish, stir applesauce, egg, milk, orange juice, orange peel, and vanilla until blended. Add to dry ingredients and stir simply until blended. Pour over cranberry mixture. Bake at 375-degree Fahrenheit (190 degree Celsius, gas mark 5) for twenty-five to 30 minutes or till picket pick inserted in the center comes out clean. Let cake cool in pan for 5 minutes. Loosen cake around the edges of the pan.
- Place inverted serving platter over the cake and turn each upside down. Shake gently, then remove the pan. Serve warm.

76 Delicious French Toast

Preparation Time: 20 minutes

Cooking Time: 15 minutes

Servings: 3

Nutritional Content Per Serving:

- Calories: 65
- Fat: 1g
- Carbohydrates: 29g
- Phosphorus: 14mg
- Potassium: 12mg
- Sodium: 09mg
- Protein: 1g

Ingredients:

- two tbsp. (25 gram) sugar
- one Loaf Low-Sodium French Bread, cut into eight Half-inches
- one mug (250 gram) egg substitute, or four eggs
- three/four mug (180 milliliters) skim milk
- one tsp. vanilla extract
- one tsp. ground cinnamon

Instructions:

- In a large mixing bowl, whisk together the eggs, milk, vanilla, and sugar. Soak the bread deeply. Remove the slices from the pan and sprinkle with cinnamon.
- Prepare on a nonstick skillet over medium heat for five to seven minutes or until golden brown on both sides.

77 Shredded Wheat Pancakes

Preparation Time: 20 minutes

Cooking Time: 15 minutes

Servings: 2

Nutritional Content Per Serving:

- Calories: 76
- Fat: 1g
- Carbohydrates: 09g
- Phosphorus: 46mg
- Potassium: 13mg
- Sodium: 11mg
- Protein: 1g

Ingredients:

- one-Half mugs (180 gram) Buttermilk Baking Mix three mugs (165 gram)
- Half mug (125 gram) egg substitute, or two eggs
- one-Half mugs (355 milliliters) skim milk
- wheat, crushed

Instructions:

- In a large mixing bowl, whisk together the eggs and milk until smooth. Incorporate the pancake mix into the batter.
- Add the shredded wheat and mix well. Allow for a five-minute rest period. Pour about a quarter mug (60 milliliters) of batter per pancake onto a nonstick skillet and cook, turning once, until golden brown, about five minutes. Twelve pancakes should suffice.

78 Gluten free Apple Oat Bran Cereal

Preparation Time: 20 minutes

Cooking Time: 15 minutes

Servings: 3

Nutritional Content Per Serving:

- Calories: 88

- Fat: 1g
- Carbohydrates: 19g
- Phosphorus: 74mg
- Potassium: 92mg
- Sodium: 47mg
- Protein: 1g

Ingredients:

- three/four mug (180 milliliters) water
- One-Fourth mug (36 gram) raisins
- Half mug (40 gram) oat bran
- Half mug (120 milliliters) apple juice
- Half tsp. ground cinnamon

Instructions:

- Mix all the ingredients in a microwave-safe dish. Microwave on high for two halves to three minutes. Serve immediately.

79 Apple Cider Cupcakes

Preparation Time: 20 minutes

Cooking Time: 40 minutes

Servings: 4

Nutritional Content Per Serving:

- Calories: 65
- Fat: 1g
- Carbohydrates: 29g
- Phosphorus: 14mg
- Potassium: 12mg
- Sodium: 17mg
- Protein: 1g

Ingredients:

- two eggs
- two mugs (220 gram) all-purpose flour
- three mugs (705 milliliters), apple cider
- one-fourth mug (165 gram) unsalted butter
- one third-fourth of mugs (350 gram) sugar

- One-Eighth tsp. ground cloves one tsp. ground cinnamon
- one tsp. sodium-free baking soda

Instructions:

- In a huge saucepan, boil the cider till it is reduced to one-Half mugs (thirty five5 milliliters) and let it cool. In a huge dish, beat together the butter and sugar with an electric mixer until it is fluffy. Beat within the eggs.
- Into the dish, sift together the flour, the cloves, the cinnamon, and the baking soda; stir in the reduced cider and mix the mixture well. Divide the batter among 18 paper-lined muffin tins and bake in the middle of a preheated 375-degree Fahrenheit (a hundred ninety-degree Celsius, gas mark 5) oven for 25 minutes, or till a tester comes out clean.

80 Hearty Scrambled Eggs with Cheese and Rice

Preparation Time: 20 minutes

Cooking Time: 40 minutes

Servings: 4

Nutritional Content Per Serving:

- Calories: 71
- Fat: 1g
- Carbohydrates: 23g
- Phosphorus: 22mg
- Potassium: 21mg
- Sodium: 21mg
- Protein: 1g

Ingredients:

- One-Fourth mug (28 gram) shredded Swiss cheddar cheese
- One-Fourth tsp. freshly ground black pepper
- one mug (165 gram) of cooked rice
- one-Half mugs (375 gram) egg substitute, or six eggs, beaten

Instructions:

- Add the rice into a skillet and pour the beaten eggs over the top. Scramble the egg until set, about five minutes. Sprinkle the cheddar cheese and pepper on top and let melt. Serve immediately.

81 Eggs with Red Onion and Spinach

Preparation Time: 20 minutes

Cooking Time: 15 minutes

Servings: 3

Nutritional Content Per Serving:

- Calories: 66
- Fat: 1g
- Carbohydrates: 20g
- Phosphorus: 31mg
- Potassium: 41mg
- Sodium: 22mg
- Protein: 1g

Ingredients:

- two tbsp. (30 milliliters) skim milk
- One-Fourth tsp. freshly ground black pepper
- five oz. (140 gram) fresh spinach
- one-Half tbsp. (21 gram) unsalted butter
- Half mug (80 gram) thinly diced red onion
- two Half mugs (625 gram) egg substitute or ten eggs

Instructions:

- Warm up the butter in a big nonstick skillet over moderate heat. Add the onion and sauté until softened, about five minutes.
- Meanwhile, in a big dish, stir together the eggs, milk, and pepper. Pour into the pan and cook, occasionally stirring, to desired doneness, four to five minutes, adding the spinach just before the eggs are set.

82 Low Sodium Grilled Asparagus

Preparation Time: 12 minutes

Cooking Time: 20 minutes

Servings: 3

Nutritional Content Per Serving:

- Calories: 74
- Fat: 1g
- Carbohydrates: 23g
- Phosphorus: 25mg
- Potassium: 27mg
- Sodium: 22mg
- Protein: 1g

Ingredients:

- one tbsp. (15 milliliters) olive oil
- one-fourth tsp. black pepper, freshly ground
- one lb. asparagus
- one tbsp. (15 milliliters) lemon juice

Instructions:

- Trim the asparagus spears and drizzle with oil and lemon juice. Season the asparagus with pepper. Grill for three to four minutes over moderately high heat, turning once the first side starts to brown in spots.

83 Mixed-Grain Hot Cereal

Preparation Time: 20 minutes

Cooking Time: 30 minutes

Servings: 3

Nutritional Content Per Serving:

- Calories: 88
- Fat: 1g
- Carbohydrates: 19g
- Phosphorus: 74mg
- Potassium: 92mg
- Sodium: 47mg
- Protein: 1g

Ingredients:

- two tbsp. uncooked whole buckwheat
- one mug peeled, diced apple
- two one-fourth mugs water
- one one-fourth mugs vanilla rice milk

- six tbsp. uncooked bulgur
- six tbsp. plain uncooked couscous
- Half tsp. ground cinnamon

Instructions:

- Heat the water and milk in a medium saucepan over medium-high heat. Toss in the bulgur, buckwheat, and apple and bring to a boil.
- Reduce the heat to low and cook for 20 to 25 minutes, or until the bulgur is soft, stirring occasionally. Remove the saucepan from the heat and add the couscous and cinnamon, stirring to combine. Enable 10 minutes to stand, wrapped, before fluffing the cereal with a fork.

84 Avocado Omelet

Preparation Time: 10 minutes

Cooking Time: 20 minutes

Servings: 3

Nutritional Content Per Serving:

- Calories: 90
- Fat: 1g
- Carbohydrates: 22g
- Phosphorus: 23mg
- Potassium: 25mg
- Sodium: 21mg
- Protein: 1g

Ingredients:

- Half avocado, peeled and diced
- One-Fourth mug (45 gram) chopped tomato
- One-Fourth mug (10 gram) alfalfa sprouts
- Half mug (125 gram) egg substitute, or two eggs
- one tbsp. (15 milliliters) water
- one tbsp. (14 gram) unsalted butter
- two tbsp. (30 gram) plain low-fat yoghurt

Instructions:

- Beat the eggs and water in a tiny dish. Add the butter to an eight-in. (twenty-cm) omelet pan and heat over moderate heat till hot. Pour in the egg mixture that should set at the perimeters directly.

- Carefully push the cooked egg to the center, tilting the pan sometimes so the uncooked egg will flow to the bottom whereas the prime stays moist. Arrange the avocado, tomato, and sprouts on half of the omelet. Fold the omelet over and flip it out onto a plate. Prime with the yoghurt.

85 Rhubarb Bread Pudding

Preparation Time: 20 minutes

Cooking Time: 13 minutes

Servings: 2

Nutritional Content Per Serving:

- Calories: 78
- Fat: 1g
- Carbohydrates: 65g
- Phosphorus: 44mg
- Potassium: 21mg
- Sodium: 18mg
- Protein: 1g

Ingredients:

- one tbsp. cornstarch
- one vanilla bean, split
- Unsalted butter for greasing the baking dish
- one-Half mugs not sweetened rice milk
- three eggs
- Half mug granulated sugar
- Ten thick pieces of white bread, cut into one-inch chunks
- two mugs chopped fresh rhubarb

Instructions:

- Warm up the oven to 350-degree Fahrenheit. Lightly grease an eight-by-eight-in. Baking dish with butter; put aside. In a big dish, stir along with the rice milk, eggs, sugar, and cornstarch. Scrape the vanilla seeds into the milk mixture and stir to blend. Add the bread to the egg mixture and stir to fully coat the bread.
- Add the chopped rhubarb and stir to combine. Let the bread and egg mixture soak for 30 minutes. Spoon the mixture into the ready baking dish, cover with aluminum foil, and bake for forty minutes. Uncover the bread pudding and bake for an additional ten minutes or until the pudding is golden brown and set. Serve heat.

86 Apple Cake

Preparation Time: 25 minutes

Cooking Time: 35 minutes

Servings: 3

Nutritional Content Per Serving:

- Calories: 89
- Fat: 1g
- Carbohydrates: 19g
- Phosphorus: 74mg
- Potassium: 91mg
- Sodium: 47mg
- Protein: 1g

Ingredients:

- two tsp. (nine gram) sodium-free baking powder
- one tsp. sodium-free baking soda
- Half tsp. ground cinnamon
- Half tsp. Ground nutmeg
- one mug (235 milliliters) vegetable oil
- two mugs (400 gram) sugar
- three eggs
- two Half mugs (275 gram) all-purpose flour
- one tsp. vanilla extract
- three mugs (450 gram) apples, peeled and chopped

Instructions:

- Combine the oil and sugar, then add the eggs. Combine flour, baking powder, baking soda, cinnamon, and nutmeg in a sifter; blend into the sugar mixture. Fold in the apples after applying the vanilla.
- Pour into a 9 x 13-inch baking tray. Bake at 350 degrees Fahrenheit (180 degrees Celsius, gas mark 4) for one to one and a half hours, or until a knife inserted in the middle comes out clean. If needed, dust the top with powdered sugar.

87 Ricotta and Spinach Omelet

Preparation Time: 20 minutes

Cooking Time: 40 minutes

Servings: 2

Nutritional Content Per Serving:

- Calories: 76
- Fat: 1g
- Carbohydrates: 15g
- Phosphorus: 74mg
- Potassium: 54mg
- Sodium: 23mg
- Protein: 1g

Ingredients:

- three tbsp. (42 gram) unsalted butter divided
- four oz. (115 gram) fresh spinach
- one mug (250 gram) egg substitute, or four eggs
- one tbsp. (15 milliliters) skim milk
- Half tsp. freshly ground black pepper
- one/three mug (83 gram) ricotta cheddar cheese

Instructions:

- Place the eggs in a very tiny mixing dish. Add the milk and pepper. Briskly stir with a fork till well crushed; set aside. In an eight-in. (20-cm) nonstick skillet, soften 2 tbsp. (twenty-eight gram) of the butter over moderate-high heat. Add the spinach and sauté till just wilted. Separate from the pan and put aside.
- Melt the remaining one tbsp. (fourteen gram) butter in the skillet, then slowly pour in the egg mixture, tilting the pan to unfold it evenly. Let the eggs firm up a little, permitting some of the remaining liquid to flow to the perimeters of the pan. Continue to cook for another minute, then spoon in the ricotta. Unfold over the omelet and prime with the spinach. Fold the opposite of the omelet over the filling.
- Shake the pan gently to slide the omelet to the edge. Holding the pan close to the serving plate, tip it so the omelet slides onto the plate.

Chapter 4: Breakfast Nuts Free

88 Nuts Free Festive Berry Parfait

Preparation Time: 10 minutes

Cooking Time: 20 minutes

Servings: 3

Nutritional Content Per Serving:

- Calories: 65
- Fat: 1g
- Carbohydrates: 11g
- Phosphorus: 71mg
- Potassium: 88mg
- Sodium: 34mg
- Protein: 1g

Ingredients:

- Half tsp. ground cinnamon
- one mug crumbled Meringue Cookies
- one mug of vanilla rice milk, at room temperature
- Half mug plain cream cheddar cheese, at room temperature
- one tbsp. granulated sugar
- two mugs, fresh blueberries
- one mug of diced fresh strawberries

Instructions:

- Stir together the milk, cream cheddar cheese, sugar, and cinnamon in a small dish until smooth. Spoon one-fourth mug of crumbled cookie into the bottom of each of four (six-ounce) containers.
- One-fourth mug of cream cheddar cheese mixture should be poured over the cookies. One-fourth mug of berries should be put on top of the cream cheddar cheese. Repeat with the cookies, cream cheddar cheese mixture, and berries in each cup.

89 Breakfast Banana Shake

Preparation Time: 10 minutes

Cooking Time: 15 minutes

Servings: 1

Nutritional Content Per Serving:

- Calories: 56
- Fat: 1g
- Carbohydrates: 11g
- Phosphorus: 17mg
- Potassium: 12mg
- Sodium: 17mg
- Protein: 1g

Ingredients:

- two tsp. instant coffee granules
- two bananas, diced and frozen (about one-Half mugs [225 gram])
- Ground cinnamon
- one mug (230 gram) low-fat vanilla frozen yoghurt
- one mug (235 milliliters) skim milk
- eight oz. (225 gram) silken tofu drained and cut into cubes

Instructions:

- Place the frozen yoghurt, milk, tofu, coffee granules, and bananas in a blender; process until smooth and frothy. Sprinkle with cinnamon, if desired.

90 Low carb Carrot-Pineapple Smoothie

Preparation Time: 20 minutes

Cooking Time: 10 minutes

Servings: 1

Nutritional Content Per Serving:

- Calories: 78
- Fat: 1g
- Carbohydrates: 29g
- Phosphorus: 24mg
- Potassium: 32mg
- Sodium: 42mg
- Protein: 1g

Ingredients:

- One-Fourth mug (28 gram) grated carrot
- Half banana
- three/four mug (124 gram) pineapple chunks
- Half mug (120 gram) ice
- one/three mug (80 milliliters) orange juice

Instructions:

- Place all the ingredients in a blender and process until smooth. Serve with the leaves of mint.

91 Cappuccino Breakfast Smoothie

Preparation Time: 20 minutes

Cooking Time: 10 minutes

Servings: 1

Nutritional Content Per Serving:

- Calories: 88
- Fat: 1g
- Carbohydrates: 19g
- Phosphorus: 74mg
- Potassium: 92mg
- Sodium: 47mg
- Protein: 1g

Ingredients:

- one tbsp. (15 gram) packed dark brown sugar
- One-Fourth tsp. Vanilla extract
- one mug (235 milliliters), skim milk
- one mug (235 milliliters), coffee
- one mug (230 gram), low-fat vanilla yoghurt
- one/eight tsp. ground cinnamon

Instructions:

- Place all the ingredients in a blender and process until smooth. Serve immediately.

92 Amazing Cooker Acorn Squash

Preparation Time: 20 minutes

Cooking Time: 10 minutes

Servings: 1

Nutritional Content Per Serving:

- Calories: 76
- Fat: 1g
- Carbohydrates: 12g
- Phosphorus: 73mg
- Potassium: 67mg
- Sodium: 37mg
- Protein: 1g

Ingredients:

- two acorn squash, halved and seeded
- three/four mug (109 gram) raisins
- three/four mug (170 gram) packed brown sugar
- one tsp. ground cinnamon
- one tsp. nutmeg
- One-Fourth mug (112 gram) unsalted butter
- Half mug (120 milliliters) water

Instructions:

- In a tiny dish, combine the brown sugar, cinnamon, and nutmeg; spoon into the squash halves. Sprinkle with the raisins. Top every with one tbsp. (14 gram) of the butter. Wrap every squash individually in heavy-duty foil; seal tightly.
- Pour water into a 5-quart (five-L) slow cooker. Place the squash, cut facet up, in the slow cooker (packets could be stacked). Cover and cook on high for four hours or till the squash is tender. Open the foil packets carefully to permit steam to escape.

93 Curried Egg Pita Pockets

Preparation Time: 20 minutes

Cooking Time: 15 minutes

Servings: 1

Nutritional Content Per Serving:

- Calories: 83
- Fat: 1g
- Carbohydrates: 11g
- Phosphorus: 72mg
- Potassium: 43mg
- Sodium: 41mg
- Protein: 1g

Ingredients:

- Half tsp. ground ginger
- two tbsp. light sour cream
- two (four-inch) plain pita bread pockets, halved
- three eggs, beaten
- one scallion, both green and white parts, finely chopped
- Half red bell pepper, finely chopped
- two tsp. unsalted butter
- one tsp. curry powder
- Half mug julienned English cucumber
- one mug roughly chopped watercress

Instructions:

- In a tiny dish, stir together the eggs, scallion, and red pepper till well blended. In a big nonstick skillet over moderate heat, soften the butter. Pour the egg mixture into the skillet and cook for concerning three minutes or till the eggs are just set, swirling the skillet, however not stirring.
- Separate the eggs from the warmth; set aside. In a little dish, stir together the curry powder, ginger, and bitter cream till well blended. Evenly split the curry sauce among the four halves of the pita bread, spreading it out on one inside edge. Divide the cucumber and watercress evenly between the halves. Spoon the eggs into the halves, dividing the mixture evenly to serve.

94 Nuts free Brownies

Preparation Time: 20 minutes

Cooking Time: 35 minutes

Servings: 2

Nutritional Content Per Serving:

- Calories: 81
- Fat: 1g
- Carbohydrates: 19g
- Phosphorus: 74mg
- Potassium: 12mg
- Sodium: 11mg
- Protein: 1g

Ingredients:

- three eggs
- Half mug (55 gram) cocoa
- third-fourth mug (83 gram) all-purpose flour
- third-fourth mug (165 gram) unsalted butter, melted
- one-Half mugs (300 gram) sugar
- one Hafts. vanilla extract
- Half tsp. sodium-free baking powder
- one mug (175 gram) chocolate chips

Instructions:

- Beat butter, sugar, vanilla, and eggs in a big dish. Mix in cocoa, flour, and baking powder. Stir to combine. Stir in chocolate chips.
- Pour into a greased nine × 13-inch pan. Bake at 350-degree Fahrenheit (180 degree Celsius, gas mark four) for 20 to 22 minutes.

95 Breakfast Salmon Patties

Preparation Time: 20 minutes

Cooking Time: 15 minutes

Servings: 1

Nutritional Content Per Serving:

- Calories: 84
- Fat: 1g
- Carbohydrates: 12g
- Phosphorus: 14mg
- Potassium: 22mg
- Sodium: 37mg
- Protein: 1g

Ingredients:

- one/three mug (55 gram) minced onion
- Half mug (60 gram) all-purpose flour
- 15 oz. (420 gram) pink salmon
- One-Fourth mug (63 gram) egg substitute, or one egg, beaten
- three tbsp. (45 milliliters) olive oil

Instructions:

- The salmon should be drained. Combine the salmon, potato, and onion in a dish until moist. Mix in the flour and divide the mixture into four patties.
- In a large skillet, heat the oil over medium heat. Fry the salmon patties for about five minutes or until golden brown.

96 New England Oatmeal

Preparation Time: 20 minutes

Cooking Time: 15 minutes

Servings: 1

Nutritional Content Per Serving:

- Calories: 68
- Fat: 1g
- Carbohydrates: 29g
- Phosphorus: 14mg
- Potassium: 12mg
- Sodium: 27mg
- Protein: 1g

Ingredients:

- two/three mug (100 gram) shredded apple
- one/three mug (50 gram) raisins
- two mugs (470 milliliters) water
- One-Fourth tsp. ground cinnamon
- one mug (80 gram) quick-cooking oats
- two tbsp. (30 milliliters) maple syrup, divided
- two tbsp. (16 gram) chopped walnuts, divided

Instructions:

- In a 2-quart (one. Eight-L) saucepan, mix the water and cinnamon; bring to a boil over moderate-high heat. Add the oats and cook for three minutes. Stir within the shredded apple, raisins, one tbsp. (15 milliliters) maple syrup, and one tbsp. (eight gram) walnuts.
- Prepare for 5 minutes longer. Divide the oatmeal between two serving bowls. Spray the remaining one tbsp. (fifteen milliliters) maple syrup over prime and sprinkle with the one tbsp. (eight gram) walnuts.

97 Nuts free Marinated Black-Eyed Peas

Preparation Time: 20 minutes

Cooking Time: 10 minutes

Servings: 2

Nutritional Content Per Serving:

- Calories: 58
- Fat: 1g
- Carbohydrates: 11g
- Phosphorus: 14mg
- Potassium: 12mg
- Sodium: 17mg
- Protein: 1g

Ingredients:

- one onion, minced
- three tbsp. (45 milliliters) red wine vinegar
- one-fourth mug (60 milliliters) olive oil
- one-Half mugs (150 gram) dried black-eyed peas
- Half mug (60 gram) red bell pepper, chopped
- one clove garlic, minced
- Half tsp. dried thyme

Instructions:

- Connect the bell peppers, garlic, and onion to the drained black-eyed peas in a medium-sized bowl. To make the marinade, mix the vinegar, olive oil, and thyme in a separate bowl.
- Pour the marinade over the black-eyed pea mixture, cover with plastic wrap, and refrigerate overnight, stirring periodically to balance the flavors.

98 Cheddar Breakfast Cookies

Preparation Time: 20 minutes

Cooking Time: 30 minutes

Servings: 4

Nutritional Content Per Serving:

- Calories: 71
- Fat: 1g
- Carbohydrates: 19g
- Phosphorus: 74mg
- Potassium: 12mg
- Sodium: 47mg
- Protein: 1g

Ingredients:

- three/four mug (90 gram) all-purpose flour
- Half tsp. sodium-free baking soda
- one-Half mugs (120 gram) quick-cooking oats
- four oz. (115 gram) Cheddar upside cheese, shredded
- two/three mug (150 gram) unsalted butter
- two/three mug (132 gram) sugar
- One-Fourth mug (63 gram) egg substitute, or one egg
- one tsp. vanilla extract
- Half mug (56 gram) wheat germ

Instructions:

- Warm up the oven to 350-degree Fahrenheit (one hundred eighty degree Celsius, or gas mark four). Grease a cookie sheet. In an exceedingly massive dish, beat along the butter, sugar, egg, and vanilla till well blended. In a very separate dish, mix the flour and baking soda; increase the butter mixture and mix well.
- Stir within the oats, cheddar cheese, and wheat germ. Drop by rounded tablespoonfuls onto the prepared cookie sheet. Bake for twelve minutes or until the edges are golden brown. Transfer to a wire cooling rack. Store in an exceedingly loosely coated container in the refrigerator or at space temperature.
-

99 Zucchini Pudding

Preparation Time: 30 minutes

Cooking Time: 20 minutes

Servings: 4

Nutritional Content Per Serving:

- Calories: 88
- Fat: 1g
- Carbohydrates: 19g
- Phosphorus: 74mg
- Potassium: 92mg
- Sodium: 47mg
- Protein: 1g

Ingredients:

- one egg
- two tbsp. (10 gram) Parmesan cheddar cheese, grated
- Half tsp. dried oregano
- , two mugs, zucchini, diced
- Half onion chopped
- two tbsp. (16 gram) all-purpose flour
- One-Eighth tsp. garlic powder

Instructions:

- In a pot of boiling water, cook the zucchini and onion until they are tender. Combine the remaining ingredients in a bowl. Toss with the vegetables.
- Preheat the oven to 350 degrees Fahrenheit (180 degrees Celsius) (180 degree Celsius, gas mark four). Fill a greased one-half-quart (one-half-L) baking pan halfway with the mixture and bake until golden brown (25 to 35 minutes).

100 Spring Squash Casserole

Preparation Time: 20 minutes

Cooking Time: 40 minutes

Servings: 2

Nutritional Content Per Serving:

- Calories: 68
- Fat: 1g
- Carbohydrates: 19g
- Phosphorus: 54mg
- Potassium: 32mg
- Sodium: 47mg
- Protein: 1g

Ingredients:

- one-fourth mug (60 gram) sour cream
- One-Eighth tsp. paprika
- two tbsp. (six gram) chives, chopped
- two mugs (230 gram), low sodium bread crumbs
- , four zucchini or yellow squash, diced
- one moderate onion, diced
- one tbsp. (14 gram) unsalted butter, melted

Instructions:

- Squash and onion should be cooked in water until almost tender. Drain the water. Combine the butter, sour cream, paprika, and chives in a mixing bowl.
- Pour in the squash that has been drained. Place in a half-quart (half-L) baking dish that has been sprayed with nonstick vegetable oil spray. Bread crumbs should be sprinkled on top. Preheat the oven to 350°F (180°C, gas mark 4) and bake for 20 minutes.

101 Sausage

Preparation Time: 20 minutes

Cooking Time: 40 minutes

Servings: 2

Nutritional Content Per Serving:

- Calories: 59
- Fat: 1g
- Carbohydrates: 19g
- Phosphorus: 24mg
- Potassium: 12mg
- Sodium: 17mg

- Protein: 1g

Ingredients:

- one-fourth tsp. mace
- Half tsp. Garlic powder
- one-fourth tsp. Onion powder
- one lb. (455 gram) pork, ground
- one-fourth tsp. Black pepper
- one-fourth tsp. White pepper
- third-fourth tsp. Dried sage
- one-fourth tsp. ground allspice

Instructions:

- Mix all mentioned ingredients, mixing well. Fry, grill, or cook on a greased baking sheet in a 325-degree Fahrenheit (170 degree Celsius, gas mark three) oven until done.

102 Special Breakfast Three Bear's Porridge

Preparation Time: 30 minutes

Cooking Time: 20 minutes

Servings: 3

Nutritional Content Per Serving:

- Calories: 75
- Fat: 1g
- Carbohydrates: 19g
- Phosphorus: 72mg
- Potassium: 12mg
- Sodium: 15mg
- Protein: 1g

Ingredients:

- one one/three mug (107 gram) quick-cooking oats
- two tbsp. (14 gram) wheat germ
- one mug (235 milliliters) skim milk
- one three/four mug (411 milliliters) water
- one tbsp. (seven gram) ground cinnamon
- One-Fourth mug (36 gram) raisins
- three tbsp. (60 gram) honey

Instructions:

- Bring the water to a boil in a very saucepan over high heat, and add the cinnamon and raisins. When the water boils, add the oats and wheat germ.
- Reduce the warmth to low and cook the porridge till all the water is absorbed and the oats are soft, 3 to five minutes. Pour the porridge into three bowls and cover every with one/three mug (eighty milliliters) milk. Dribble one tbsp. (20 gram) honey over each bowlful.

103   Egg-In-The-Hole

Preparation Time: 20 minutes

Cooking Time: 30 minutes

Servings: 2

Nutritional Content Per Serving:

- Calories: 58
- Fat: 1g
- Carbohydrates: 19g
- Phosphorus: 74mg
- Potassium: 22mg
- Sodium: 17mg
- Protein: 1g

Ingredients:

- two eggs
- two tbsp. chopped fresh chives
- Pinch cayenne pepper
- two (Half-inch-thick) slices of Italian bread
- one-fourth mug unsalted butter
- Freshly ground black pepper

Instructions:

- Using a cookie cutter or a tiny glass, cut a 2-inch spherical from the center of every piece of bread. In a big nonstick skillet over moderate-high heat, soften the butter. Place the bread in the skillet, toast it for one minute, and then flip the bread over.
- Crack the eggs into the holes in the middle of the bread and cook for two minutes or till the eggs are set, and the bread is golden brown. Top with chopped chives, cayenne pepper, and black pepper. Prepare the bread for another 2 minutes. Transfer an egg-in-the-hole to each plate to serve.

104 Breakfast Rocky Road Pizza

Preparation Time: 20 minutes

Cooking Time: 30 minutes

Servings: 3

Nutritional Content Per Serving:

- Calories: 78
- Fat: 1g
- Carbohydrates: 19g
- Phosphorus: 34mg
- Potassium: 42mg
- Sodium: 37mg
- Protein: 1g

Ingredients:

- one-Half mugs (165 gram) all-purpose flour
- one one-fourth mugs (215 gram) chocolate chips
- one half mugs miniature marshmallows
- third-fourth mug (165 gram) unsalted butter
- third-fourth mug (170 gram) brown sugar
- one egg yolk
- one tsp. vanilla extract
- Half mug (75 gram) unsalted dry-roasted peanuts, chopped

Instructions:

- Beat the butter in a massive mixing dish with an electric mixer at moderate to high speed for thirty seconds. Add brown sugar and beat until combined. Beat in egg yolk and vanilla till combined. Beat in as much of the flour as you'll be able to with the mixer. Stir in any remaining flour with a picket spoon.
- Spread dough in a gently greased twelve-inch (thirty-cm) pizza pan. Bake during a 350-degree Fahrenheit (180 degree Celsius, gas mark four) oven for 25 minutes or till golden. Sprinkle hot crust with the chocolate pieces. Let stand one to two minutes to melt. Spread chocolate over crust. Sprinkle with marshmallows and nuts. Bake three minutes a lot of or till marshmallows are puffed and beginning to brown. Cool in pan on a wire rack.

105 Swiss Corn Bake

Preparation Time: 20 minutes

Cooking Time: 30 minutes

Servings: 2

Nutritional Content Per Serving:

- Calories: 68
- Fat: 1g
- Carbohydrates: 19g
- Phosphorus: 14mg
- Potassium: 12mg
- Sodium: 27mg
- Protein: 1g

Ingredients:

- two eggs
- , two tbsp. (20 gram) onion, minced
- 16 oz. (455 gram) frozen corn
- six oz. (175 milliliters) evaporated skim milk
- three oz. (85 gram) Swiss cheddar cheese, shredded, divided
- one mug (115 gram) low sodium bread crumbs

Instructions:

- Mix corn, milk, about a third-fourth of the cheddar cheese, eggs, and onion. Place in a ten × six-inch greased baking dish. Mix bread crumbs with remaining cheddar cheese.
- Sprinkle on top. Bake at 350-degree Fahrenheit (180 degree Celsius, gas mark four) for 25 to 30 minutes.

106 Breakfast-Style Grilled Cheese Sandwich

Preparation Time: 30 minutes

Cooking Time: 20 minutes

Servings: 2

Nutritional Content Per Serving:

- Calories: 66
- Fat: 1g
- Carbohydrates: 19g
- Phosphorus: 14mg
- Potassium: 22mg

- Sodium: 17mg
- Protein: 1g

Ingredients:

- 3tsp. unsalted butter, at room temperature, divided
- four Slices Low-Sodium Whole Wheat Bread two oz. (55 gram)
- Half mug (125 gram) egg substitute, or two eggs
- two tbsp. (30 milliliters) skim milk
- One-Fourth tsp. freshly ground black pepper
- Swiss cheddar cheese
- four slices low-sodium bacon, cooked

Instructions:

- Beat the eggs, milk, and pepper in a dish until blended. Heat one tsp. of the butter during a big nonstick skillet over moderate heat till hot.
- Pour in the egg mixture. As the eggs begin to set, unfold into a thin layer and cook, pull, lift, fold the eggs, till thickened and no visible liquid egg remains. Separate from the pan and clean the skillet. Spread the remaining 2 tsp. butter evenly on one aspect of each slice of bread. Place two slices in the skillet, buttered facet down. Top evenly with the scrambled eggs, cheddar cheese, and bacon.
- Cover with the remaining two slices of bread, buttered facet up. Grill the sandwiches over moderate heat, turning once, till the bread is toasted and the cheddar cheese is melted, two to four minutes.

107 Devil's Food Cake

Preparation Time: 30 minutes

Cooking Time: 20 minutes

Servings: 2

Nutritional Content Per Serving:

- Calories: 79
- Fat: 1g
- Carbohydrates: 12g
- Phosphorus: 12mg
- Potassium: 13mg
- Sodium: 19mg
- Protein: 1g

Ingredients:

- one tbsp. (14 gram) sodium-free baking soda
- two-third mug (147 gram) applesauce one-third mug (80 milliliters) buttermilk
- two tbsp. vegetable oil
- two mugs (220 gram) all-purpose flour
- one third-fourth of mugs (350 gram) sugar
- Half mug (55 gram) not sweetened cocoa powder
- one mug (235 milliliters) of coffee

Instructions:

- Warm-up oven to 350-degree Fahrenheit (a hundred and eighty degree Celsius, gas mark four). Spray a) pan with nonstick vegetable oil spray and then dirt with flour, shaking out the excess. In a huge dish, combine flour, sugar, cocoa, and baking soda. Stir within the applesauce, buttermilk, and oil.
- Warm-up coffee to boiling. Stir into batter. The mixture can be thin. Pour into pan. Bake 35 to forty minutes until a toothpick inserted in the middle comes out clean.

108 Breakfast Pizzas

Preparation Time: 20 minutes

Cooking Time: 30 minutes

Servings: 4

Nutritional Content Per Serving:

- Calories: 56
- Fat: 1g
- Carbohydrates: 11g
- Phosphorus: 33mg
- Potassium: 53mg
- Sodium: 13mg
- Protein: 1g

Ingredients:

- Half mug (125 gram) egg substitute, or two eggs, beaten
- One-Fourth mug (28 gram) shredded Swiss cheddar cheese
- two tbsp. (33 gram) Low-Sodium Spaghetti Sauce

Instructions:

- In an oven or toaster oven, preheat the broiler and place the oven rack six inches (15 cm) below the heat source.

- Cook over moderate-high heat in a small skillet coated with cooking spray. Cook, frequently stirring, until the eggs are set, one to two minutes. On the English muffin halves, spread the sauce. Scrambled egg and cheddar cheese on top.

APPETIZERS & BEVERAGES

109 APPLE BRIE AND ARUGULA PIZZA WITH HONEY

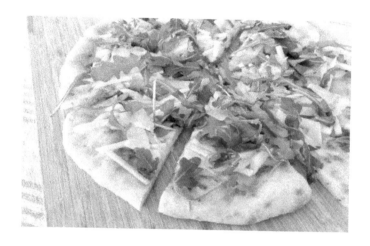

This pizza is bright and delicious. It's perfect pizza to enjoy in summer or spring!

Preparation time: 15 minutes

Cooking time: 10 minutes

Serving: 4

INGREDIENTS
- 1 batch pizza paste
- Corn stack to sprinkle
- 2 tablespoons of olive oil
- Salt
- 4 ounces mozzarella shredded

- 4 ounces brie cut into strips; strings garnished
- 1 small honey Crisp or your favorite Sweet-Ish, Part-Ish apple
- 1/2 lemon
- 2 cups of cool rocket
- 1/4 cup shaved parmesan
- Honey for drizzling

INSTRUCTIONS

➤ Preheat the oven to 550F. If you have a pizza stone, place the stone in the oven while preheating and better results, let it sit in the hot oven about 30 minutes before making the pizza.

➤ If you have a pizza peel, on a large sheet of parchment paper, sprinkle a generous amount of corn. If you do not have pizza peel, sprinkle the corn on the entire cooking sheet you cook the pizza. Use your hands to stretch the pizza dough until it is a 12-inch circle. It's good if it's not a perfect circle, mine is definitely never! Place the circle on your cooking sheet or parchment paper. Let it rest for a few minutes while you prepare the apple.

➤ Peel the apple, remove the kernel and cut it into thin matt. Mix the apple sticks in a bowl with 1/2 lemon juice and set aside.

➤ Brush the dough with olive oil until all the dough has been brushed with oil. Make sure you do not put as much oil on the pizza it sets up in places, otherwise the pizza will become too fat. You can use more or less than the 2 tablespoons, it goes to the ocular globe a bit.

➤ Sprinkle salt on the dough. Then sprinkle mozzarella uniformly on the dough, leaving a border for the crust. Uniformly distribute the slices of brie on the pizza.

- Transfer the pizza to the oven, on the pizza stone if you have one. If you cook on a pizza stone, the pizza will cook a little faster, in about 5-6 minutes. If you do not have a stone, it will cook in about 7-9 minutes. Make sure to keep an eye on the pizza, the oven is really hot so that it will cook quickly! Once the crust has slightly golden and swollen and the cheese browned a little, remove the oven.

- Leave the cool pizza for 5 minutes, then high with the Apple matches. Sprinkle uniformly the rocket on the pizza, then garnish with fresh rocket. Sprinkle the shaved parmesan on the pizza, and went up with a very brunet of honey on the whole pie.

- Slicer, serve and enjoy!

110 BAKED GARLIC

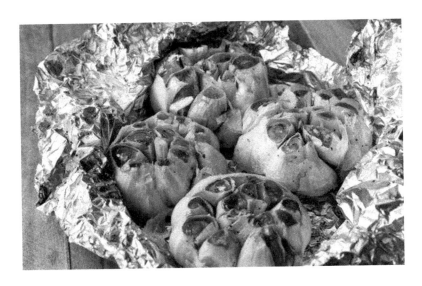

Preparation time: 5mins

Total time: 45mins

Serves about 10

1 serving = about 7-8 pods

INGREDIENTS

- 1 big head of garlic
- Extra virgin olive oil
- Kosher salt
- Black pepper freshly ground

DIRECTION

➢ Preheat the oven to 400 °. Slice from the top of the head of garlic. Sprinkle oil and season with salt and pepper. Wrap in sheet and place in a shallow dish.

> Roast to Golden and sweet, 40 minutes. Let cool then tighten the garlic cloves and use everything.

111 BROCCOLI DIP IN FRENCH BREAD

Preparation time: 10 mins

Cooking time: 25mins

Servings: Pre serve

INGREDIENTS

- 1 package (10 ounces) frozen chopped broccoli
- 1 mug dairy sour cream
- 1 mug of mayonnaise
- 2 table spoons of chopped green onions, including high
- 2 tablespoons chopped parsley
- 1 JAR (2 ounces) Diced Pimiento, drained
- 1/2 teaspoon of dill weed
- 1/4 teaspoon salt
- 1/8 Coffee spoon of garlic powder
- 1 French bread

INSTRUCTIONS

Thaw broccoli; Press the excess moisture with a paper towel. Cut finely broccoli. In a small bowl, combine the sour cream and mayonnaise; Mix well. Incorporate the broccoli and the remaining ingredients except bread. Refrigerate at least 2 hours to mix flavors. Slice the superior crust of the French bread; hollow inside the bread. Cut the bread removed into pieces; Place the pieces on a sheet of ungreased cookies. Cook in 350 ° F. oven for 8 to 10 minutes or until slightly grilled. The spoon plunges the spoon into bread. Garnish as you wish. Serve with pieces of toast, crackers or vegetable bushes.

NUTRITIONAL INFORMATION

Servings: 32 (2 tablespoons of each), Size of service: per serving, Calories: 61, Cholesterol: 5 mg, FAT: 6 g, Sodium: 69 mg, Carbohydrates: 1 g

112 DEVILED EGGS

Prep:15

Serving: 12

INGREDIENTS
+ Paprika's dash
+ Pepper
+ 2 tablespoons. (30 ml) Mayonnaise
+ ½ tsp. (2.5 ml) Dry mustard
+ ½ tsp. (2.5 ml) vinegar
+ 1 tablespoon. (15 ml) onion, finely chopped
+ 4 hard eggs

INSTRUCTIONS
> Cut the eggs in half the length and remove the yellow.

- ➤ Mash Yolks with a fork and mix with
- ➤ Remaining ingredients (except paprika).
- ➤ Reload eggs, pinging slightly.
- ➤ Sprinkle with paprika.
- ➤ Serves 4
- ➤ 1 serving (2 pieces) = 1 meat and choice of meat

113 Mexican nibbles

Cooking time: 15 mins

Preparation time: 10 mins

Serving: 1

Total time: 30 mins

INGREDIENTS
- 1 white egg, ambient temperature
- 2½ tsp. chili powder
- ½ tsp. cumin
- ¼ c. garlic powder
- 3 cups of Cereal® Cereal life or another square cereal of corn

INSTRUCTIONS
Beat the egg white until frothy. Combine 3 following ingredients in bowl, mix well; Fold in a white egg. Add cereals, stir gently to coat. Spread the mixture on a slightly greased cookie sheet. Cook 325 ° F for 15 minutes, stirring every 5 minutes. Cool on the sheet.

Strictly covered store.

Made 6 cups

114 NUTS & BOLTS SNACK MIX

Prep time: 10 mins

Cook time: 2hours

Serving: 32

Total time: 2 hours 10 mins

INGREDIENTS

- 4 cups Chex cereals or shred dies
- 3 cups of cheerios cereals
- 3 cups of pretzel sticks
- 2 cups of small pretzels
- 1 cup of small simple crackers (1 to 1 1/2-inch size, use cheese flavored crackers, if you wish)
- 2 cups of roasted salty peanuts
- 1 cup of pecans (optional)
- 1 cup of non-salted butter (melted)
- 1 1/2 teaspoon of garlic powder
- 1 teaspoon of onion powder
- 2 tablespoons of Worcestershire sauce
- 1 teaspoon of smoked paprika
- 1 1/2 to 2 teaspoons of seasoning salt
- a pinch of Sriracha or another hot sauce (optional, for non-spictious flavor)

INSTRUCTIONS

- ➢ Turn your slow cooker and add cereals, pretzels, crackers and nuts.
- ➢ In a small bowl, combine melted butter, garlic, onion powder, unemployed sauce, paprika, seasoning salt and Sriracha. A small tip of Sriracha will not make the spicy snack mix, it just adds a flavor.
- ➢ Pour the butter mixture on the ingredients of the slow cooker and mix softly but carefully with a rubber spatula (this prevents the ingredients from breaking up) until everything is well coated.
- ➢ Story on your stove slow for about 2 hours, stirring every half hour. I recommend taking the lid of the slowness for the last 15 minutes of cooking to leave a moisture evaporate.
- ➢ Make sure to leave the snack mix to cool completely before packing for storage in a hermetic container. This will prevent the snack mixture from Soggy and keep it well and crisp. The best way to do it is on a parchment paper on a large tray or a pastry plate.
- ➢ Once the snack mixture is completely cooled, store it in waterproof containers or serve immediately.

"Prepare this snack mix until a week in advance and store it in hermetic containers to serve you later.

This snack mix can also be baked for about 4 hours, stirring every hour".

Nutrition

Serve: 0.5cup | Calories: 197kcal | Carbohydrates: 17g | Protein: 5G | FAT: 13G | Saturated grease: 5g | Cholesterol: 15mg | Sodium: 347mg | Potassium: 133mg | Fiber: 2G | Sugar: 1G | Vitamin A: 400iU | Vitamin C: 2mg | Calcium: 39mg | Iron: 3mg

115 SAY CHEESE RECIPE

Preparation time: 30 mins

Cooking time: 37

Serving: 4 to 6

INGREDIENTS

- 1 tablespoon of non-salty butter
- 1 big cauliflower head (about 2 pounds)
- 4 1/2 ounces cheddar, grated and divided
- 1/2 cup of crude bread crumbs made house
- 1 whole egg
- 1 teaspoon of salt kosher
- 1 teaspoon of dry mustard powder
- 1/2 Smoked Paprika Coffee Spoon
- 1/4 teaspoon of black pepper freshly ground
- 1/4 Cayenne pepper teaspoon
- 1/2 cup of thick cream

INSTRUCTIONS

- ➢ Grease a 7-inch flame cooking dish with butter and set aside.
- ➢ Position 1 oven grill in the central position and 1 in the upper position and preheat the oven to 400 degrees F.
- ➢ Place the cauliflower in a small glass bowl, the stem finishes. Use a paring knife to eliminate the lower leaves. Cut the clots of the stem, keeping them as intact as possible. Try keeping the size uniformly large and do so few cuts as possible. Discard the leaves and the stem. Cover tightly with a plastic film

and a high-pressure microwave for 4 minutes. Rest, always covered with plastic, for more 4 minutes. Discover and rest for 4 to 5 minutes more while preparing the rest of the dish.

➤ Combine 4 ounces of cheese, crumbs of bread, egg, salt, mustard, paprika, black pepper and cayenne in a large bowl to mix. When a minute stays on the rest period of the cauliflower, microwave the high cream for 30 seconds. Add the cream to the bowl with the cheese mix and mix to combine.

➤ Using your hands and tea towel if the cauliflower is still hot, rub the big florets in your hands to break the clots. Add the clots to the cream mixture and stir until the cheese is carefully melted and combined.

➤ Spread the cauliflower blend in the prepared cookware, place it on the middle rack and cook for 20 minutes. Remove the baking dish and turn the chicken to the hen sprinkle the rest of the 1/2 oz cheese at the top of the cauliflower. Place on the upper rack and grill until the top is bubble and brown appropriately, 6 to 8 minutes. Refills 10 minutes before serving.

116 STRAWBERRY- LEMONADE SLUSH

INGREDIENTS
+ 12 Washed strawberries and hulls
+ 1 Campaign time lemonade cup
+ 5 cups of water
+ Sprite or ginger-ale

Preparation time: 8 mins

Serving: 8

INSTRUCTIONS

- ➢ Using a culinary mixer or robot, mashed strawberries.
- ➢ Pour into a large bowl.
- ➢ Add to the mixture and water and stir until dissolving the lemonade mixture.
- ➢ Pour into a plate of 9 × 13 (plastic or metal) and place in the freezer.
- ➢ Define a timer for 1 hour.
- ➢ Mix of scrap with a fork. It will always be liquid enough, but ice crystals should form on top and around the edges.
- ➢ Repeat every hour for 4 hours, shift and stir the mixture.
- ➢ Once all that is broken and looks like shaved ice, scoop about 1 cup of the silhouette to a cup and fill it with sprite or ginger.
- ➢ To serve.
- ➢ Can be done 2 weeks in advance. Keep in an airtight container in the freezer Ù

117 WONTON SOUP WITH ANIS STAR BROTH

Is an easy recipe from the Wonton soup, made with frozen wontons and a deep broth and rich soy sauce, star anise, cinnamon, ginger and garlic?

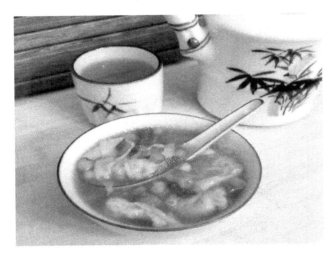

Preparation time: 10 minutes

Cooking time: 1 hour

Total time: 1 hour 10 minutes

Servings: 6 people

INGREDIENTS
+ 8 cups of chicken broth
+ 3 tablespoons soy sauce
+ 4 tablespoons of chopped fresh ginger
+ 4 cloves of garlic
+ Anise 3 stars
+ 1 cinnamon stick
+ 2 Thai peppers
+ 30 WOONTONS
+ 4 Sliced Green Onions

INSTRUCTIONS

- In a big pot, bring the broth, soy sauce, ginger, garlic, star anise, cinnamon and chilies to a boil. Cook with a low boil for 45 minutes.
- Suffer the broth, throwing ginger, garlic, star anise, cinnamon stick and peppers.
- Bring to a small boil and throw in the Wontons. Cook for another 10 minutes.
- Serve in sprinkling bowls some green onions on the top of the soup.

118 WALNUT TACOS WITH PEACH SALSA

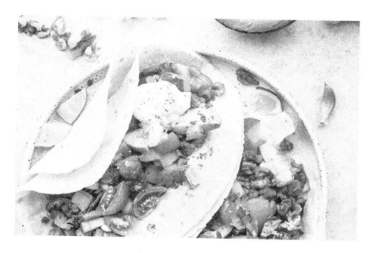

Preparation time: 15 mins

Cooking time: 5mins

Serving: 4

INGREDIENT
- 2Whole walnut cups
- 1 ½ Smoked paprika at the TSER
- ½ cumin
- 1 ½ Pint powder at c.
- ½ little spoon of salt

- 1 Water soup spoon
- 1 Soup spoon of lemon juice
- 1 Great fishing, finely ubicated
- 1Red pepper, finely cut into dice
- 1 pint of cherry tomatoes, half
- 1 Garlic clove, mined
- salt and pepper
- 1 lawyer
- ¼ chopped red cabbage cup
- ¼ Simple yogurt cut or optional sour cream
- lime juice

INSTRUCTION

> Pulse the nuts in a culinary robot until finely collapsed, four or five times (be careful not to pulse!).
> Transfer of paprika, chili and cumin into a saucepan over medium heat and toast for 30 seconds, stirring often. Add nuts and salt and launch. Add water and lime juice and stir up to completely coated. Remove from heat and set aside.
> Add all the ingredients of salsa in a bowl and mix to combine. Season with salt and pepper.
> Reheat the tortillas in a saucepan over medium heat for 10 seconds. Doubling tortillas and place 1/4 of nuts and fishing salsa. Repeat with the remaining tortillas. Top with lawyer, cabbage and yogurt or sour cream (if you use). Serve hot.
>

DESSERTS

119 CHINESE ALMOND COOKIES

Preparation: 20 minutes
Cook: 15 minutes
Serving: 48

INGREDIENTS
- ❖ 1 cup of softened butter at room temperature
- ❖ 1 cup of sugar
- ❖ 1 egg
- ❖ 1 1/2 teaspoon of almond extract
- ❖ 1 teaspoon of cooking powder
- ❖ 1/2 teaspoon salt
- ❖ 3 cups of all-purpose flour
- ❖ 1 beaten white egg with 1 tablespoon of water
- ❖ 2 tablespoons of sliced almonds

INSTRUCTIONS
- ➢ Preheat the oven to 325 degrees.
- ➢ In a large cream bowl set butter and sugar until light and mellow. Beat in 1 egg, almond extract, cooking powder and salt. Add slowly into the 3 cups of flour. Beat until the dough is well mixed. Divide the dough into 1 inch balls, it's very easy to do with a cookie spoon.
- ➢ Place the 2-inch interval dough balls on a non-greased pastry plate. Aplace pulp balls with the bottom of a glass. Brush the top of the cookies with the white washing of the eggs and sprinkle almond slices on the top of the biscuit.

> Cook the cookie for 12 to 14 minutes or until the cookie begins to become golden brown. Transfer the cookies to a wire holder and let yourself be cooled completely before storing in a hermetic container.

NUTRITION
Calories: 82kcal | Carbohydrates: 10g | Protein: 1G | FAT: 4G | Saturated grease: 2G | Cholesterol: 13mg | Sodium: 60mg | Potassium: 23mg | Fiber: 0g | Sugar: 4G | Vitamin A: 125iu | Calcium: 8mg | Iron: 0.4 m

120 CRANBERRY COOKIE KISSES

Preparation: 10 minutes
Cook: 2 hr
Serving: 20

INGRENDIENT
- ❖ 3 big egg white, at room temperature
- ❖ ¼ tsp. Tartar cream.
- ❖ ¾ sugar cup.
- ❖ ¼ cup canned cranberry sauce, all berries
- ❖ 1/3 cup of dry cranberry, around 80 cranberries

INSTRUCTIONS
> Heat the oven to 200 ° F. Coat 2 large cake sheet pans with cooking spray with parchment paper.
> Use a mixture of electricity, shake egg white and cream Tartar until a rigid peak is formed; gradually defeat sugar until the mixture is very stiff and sparkling. Stir Cranberry Sauce (You can add a few drops of red food dyes on this point, if desired); Beat for 1 minute.
> Drop the mixture with a teaspoon to the prepared sheet pan; Press 1 Cranberry Dry to the top of each cookie.

- ➤ Bake for about 2 hours, turn off the oven afterwards 15 minutes. It's cool completely before taking off from the pan.
- ➤ Save Cookies in an airtight container.

121 CRANBERRY DIP WITH FRESH FRUIT

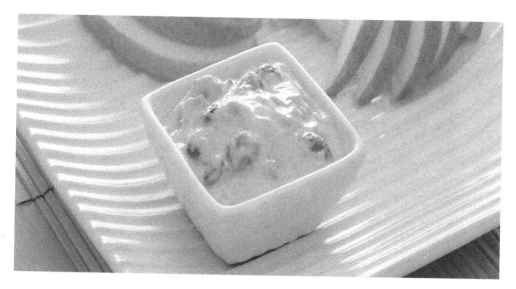

Preparation: 10 minutes
Cook: 1hours
Serving: 24

INGREDIENTS
- ❖ 8 ounces sour cream
- ❖ ½ cup of entire bay cranberry sauce
- ❖ ¼ c. Nutmeg
- ❖ ¼ c. grounded ginger
- ❖ 4 medium apples, cut in 12 slices each
- ❖ Canned pears, 12 slices
- ❖ 4 cup fresh pineapple, cut into cut pieces
- ❖ lemon juice

INSTRUCTIONS

- ➢ Place the sour cream, cranberry sauce, nutmeg
- ➢ and ginger in a culinary robot and a process
- ➢ Until well mixed. Delete in a small bowl.
- ➢ Cut the fresh fruits into size pieces.
- ➢ Mix the apple with lemon juice to prevent browning.
- ➢ Organize fruit on a tray with a bowl in the
- ➢ middle. Cool until it is ready to serve.

NUTRIENTS

Calories 70, protein 0 g, carbohydrates 13 g, grease 2 g, cholesterol 4 mg, sodium 8 mg, potassium 101 mg, phosphorus 15 mg, calcium 17 mg, 1,5 g fiber

122 CRANBERRY PINEAPPLE LOAF

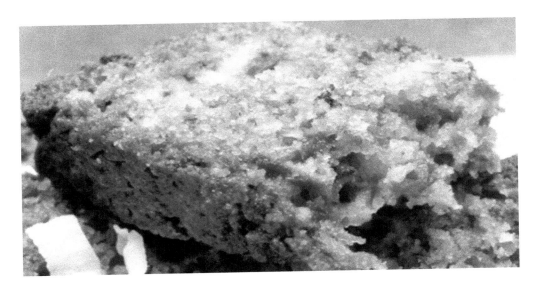

Preparation: 10 minutes
Cook: 1hrs 10 mins
Serving: 14

INGREDIENTS

- ❖ 3 best eggs from Auber glands
- ❖ 1 cup of canola oil
- ❖ 2 cups of granulated sugar

- ❖ 12 oz cranberry bag
- ❖ 1 8oz. Can be crushed pineapple (drained)
- ❖ 3 cups of flour
- ❖ 2 c. Soda bicarbonate tea
- ❖ 1/2 c. Cooking powder
- ❖ 1 C. TSP salt
- ❖ 1/2 muscade nut teaspoon
- ❖ 1/2 ginger teaspoon
- ❖ 1/2 cinnamon teaspoon

PREPARATION

- ➢ Preheat the oven to 350 degrees; Coat two 9-inch bread rolls with an anti-adhesive cooking aerosol.
- ➢ Pulse cranberries in a culinary robot to cut; put aside.
- ➢ Tie together the flour, baking soda, cooking powder, salt, cinnamon, ginger and nutmeg set and set aside.
- ➢ With an electric mixer, beat eggs, oil and sugar for 3 minutes at average speed. Stir in chopped cranberries and crushed pineapple.
- ➢ Add dry ingredients to wet ingredients; Incorporate just enough to combine mixtures - do not overcome too much.
- ➢ Divide the mixture uniformly into the two pans; Cook for 1 hour and 10 minutes, or until a knife inserted in the middle exits clean.

NUTRIENT

Calories 225, Grease 10g (39% fat calories), 32g cholesterol, sodium 213 mg, 32g carbohydrates, 1G food fiber, 3G protein.

BEEF

123 BEEF AND BARLEY STEW

Preparation: 20 minutes

Cook: 1hr

Serving: 8

INGREDIENTS:
- ❖ 2 tablespoons of olive oil
- ❖ 1 1/2 pounds of upper swirl steak, diced
- ❖ Kosher salt and freshly ground black pepper, to taste
- ❖ 1 medium sweet onion, diced
- ❖ 3 medium carrots, peeled and diced
- ❖ 2 celery ribs, dice cut
- ❖ 3 garlic cloves, minced
- ❖ 2 cups of sliced mushrooms
- ❖ 1/3 cup of red or dry white wine
- ❖ 8 cups of beef stock
- ❖ 1 cup of beaded barley, rinsed
- ❖ 5 Sprigs Thyme Fresh
- ❖ 1 bay sheet
- ❖ 2 tablespoons of chopped fresh parsley leaves

DIRECTIONS:
- ➢ Heating olive oil in a large stock or a medium heat. Season steak with salt and pepper, to taste. Add to the stockout and cook, stirring from time to time until it is uniformly golden, about 6-8 minutes; put aside.
- ➢ Add the onion, carrots and celery. Cook, stirring occasionally, until tender, about 3-4 minutes.
- ➢ Add garlic and fungi and cook from time to time, until tender and gold, about 3-4 minutes.

- Stir in the wine, scratching golden bits from the bottom of the stock.
- Incorporate the stock of beef, barley, thyme, bay sheet and steak. Bring to a boil; Reduce heat and simmer, covered until barley is tenderness, about 45 minutes. Remove and discard the thyme twigs and the bay sheet. Incorporate parsley; Season with salt and pepper according to your taste. *
- Seers immediately.
-

124 BEEF KABOBS

Preparation: 2Hrs
Cook: 10 mins
Serving: 4

INGREDIENTS

- ❖ 1 pound beef sirloin
- ❖ ½ cup of vinegar
- ❖ 2 tablespoons. salad oil
- ❖ 1 medium onion, chopped
- ❖ 2 tablespoons. chopped fresh parsley
- ❖ ¼ c. black pepper
- ❖ 2 green peppers, cut in broad bands

INSTRUCTIONS

Cut the fat from the meat. Cut into cubes of 1 ½ ".

- ➢ Mix vinegar, oil, onion, parsley and pepper. Marinate Meat in a mixture for 2 hours stirring occasionally.
- ➢ Remove the meat from the marinade and alternate 4 skewers with green pepper. Brush with marinade.
- ➢ 4 inches grill of heat about 10 minutes, turning once.

Note: If you do not have skewers, the Kabob Shish

- ➢ The ingredients can be grills in a saucepan. Follow the steps 1 and 2 above. Sprinkle a few c. marinade on vegetables and grills until tender, stirring once.

NUTRIENT

1 portion = 3 proteins, 1 low potassium vegetable

125 CONFETTI RICE

Preparation: 20 mins
Cook: 10 mins
Serving: 6

INGREDIENTS

- ❖ 1 book (454 g) lean chopped beef
- ❖ 1 c. Margarine
- ❖ 1 cup of rice, white, long grain, raw
- ❖ 2 cups of beef broth, reduced sodium
- ❖ 1 ½ cup frozen mixed vegetables
- ❖ 1 ½ tablespoon. Seasoning with garlic and herbs (Ms. Dash or McCormick's no added salt)

INSTRUCTIONS

- ➢ In a large frying pan, the brown beef drinks in the middle Heat until no pink color remains. Empty fat.
- ➢ Incorporate seasoning with garlic and grass and margarine.
- ➢ Incorporate raw rice, add beef broth.
- ➢ Let the blend with a medium heat. Turn heat to Low, lid stove with lid and simmer about 10 minutes.
- ➢ Remove the lid; mix well. Add frozen vegetables and mix
- ➢ Once again, (if the mixture is dry, add a small amount of water).
- ➢ Coverage. Simmer still 5-10 minutes until rice and the vegetables are cooked.

NUTRIENT

1 portion = 3 proteins, 2 starch, 1 average potassium.

126 CRANBERRY MEATLOAF

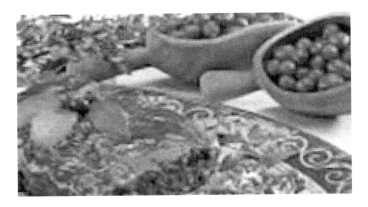

Preparation: 20 mins
Cook: 1 Hrs.
Serving: 5

INGREDIENTS

- ❖ 1 lb lean chopped beef
- ❖ ½ cup bread breadcrumbs or not salaried cracker bumps
- ❖ 2 eggs
- ❖ 1 ½ tsp. lemon juice
- ❖ 2 tsp. dried mustard
- ❖ 1/3 cup jelly cranberry sauce

INSTRUCTIONS

Prepare the oven at 350 ° F. Combine all the ingredients in a bread form. Place in a slightly greased pan.

NUTRIENT

1 servant = 3 proteins, 1 starch

127 IRISH STEW

Preparation: 20 mins
Cook: 3 Hrs.
Serving: 4

INGREDIENTS

- ❖ 10 ounces (300g) beef cubes
- ❖ 1 tablespoon. oil
- ❖ 2 finely chopped onions
- ❖ 1 clove garlic, mined
- ❖ 1 ½ cup of weak sodium beef broth
- ❖ ½ cup of sliced carrots, boiled *
- ❖ 1 cup of potatoes, cubes and boiled *
- ❖ 1 bay sheet
- ❖ ½ tsp. Rosemary
- ❖ 1/8 TSP. pepper
- ❖ ½ tsp. parsley

INSTRUCTIONS

- ➤ Cubes of brown beef in ½ tablespoon. oil. Remove from the pan.
- ➤ Cooking with garlic and onion in the remaining oil until brown.
- ➤ Add a broth and seasonings; Cover and simmer for an hour.
- ➤ Add vegetables; Bake until the stew is full heated.

* If you follow a low potassium diet, you can decrease the potassium content soaking them in the water for at least 4 hours or double bubbling (do not save water).

1 serving = 2 protein, 1 medium potassium vegetable

128 ITALIAN MEATBALLS WITH PARSLEY AND PARMESAN

Preparation: 20 mins
Cook: 35 mins.
Serving: 10

INGREDIENTS

- ❖ 4 big eggs (or 1 cup of egg drummers)
- ❖ ½ cup of fresh breadcrumbs
- ❖ 6 c. Parmesan cheese
- ❖ 3 c. olive oil
- ❖ ¼ cup fresh parsley and chopped fresh
- ❖ 3 large cloves of garlic, peeled and sliced
- ❖ 1 medium onion, chopped
- ❖ 1 tablespoon. Dijon's mustard
- ❖ 1 C. black pepper
- ❖ 2 pounds of lean chopped beef

INSTRUCTIONS

- ➤ Incorporate eggs, bread crumbs, parmesan cheese, olive oil, onion, Parsley, garlic, mustard and pepper in a big bowl.
- ➤ Add chopped beef and mix thoroughly.
- ➤ Form the mixture in 1 ½ "diameter balls.
- ➤ Spray a cookie sheet with cooking sprayer (WFP).
- ➤ Place the meatballs on a single-layer cookie sheet.
- ➤ Cook at 350 ° F for 30 to 40 minutes, or until brown.

1 serving = 4 meatball = 3 choice of proteins

129 MEATBALLS WITH ROASTED RED PEPPER SAUCE

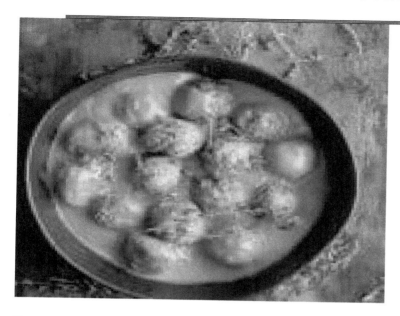

Preparation: 15 mins
Cook: 15 mins.
Serving: 24

INGREDIENTS

- ❖ 3 lb of chopped beef
- ❖ 4 big eggs or 1 cup of egg drummers
- ❖ ¾ cup of fresh breadcrumbs
- ❖ 6 c. Parmesan cheese
- ❖ 1 tablespoon. olive oil
- ❖ 1 tablespoon. Garlic powder or 3 large cloves of garlic, peeled and chinned
- ❖ 2 tsp. Oregano dried
- ❖ 1 cup of onion, minced
- ❖ 1 C. ground black pepper

INSTRUCTIONS

- ➢ Preheat the oven to 375 ° F
- ➢ Combine all the ingredients in a large bowl and mix together.
- ➢ Roll in 1 "bullets and places it on a pastry plate.
- ➢ Cook for 10-15 minutes until meatballs are cooked.

> Serve, place meatballs in a heating dish or a rider pot on low Heat. Serve with 2 TSP. sauce. (See sauce recipe)

1 serving = 2 meatballs = 3 proteins

130 ROASTED RED PEPPER SAUCE

Preparation: 5 mins
Cook: 30 mins.
Serving: 16

INGREDIENTS
- ❖ 2 roasted whole red peppers
- ❖ 1-2 clove garlic, minced
- ❖ 1 C. olive oil
- ❖ 1 C. Dried Italian seasonings (no added salt)
- ❖ ¼ cup of red pepper chili flakes (if the spicy desire)

INSTRUCTIONS
> Roasted pepper in the grill or barbecue until the skin becomes black. Pepper Cool, then take off the skin and throw. Puree peppers, garlic, black Pepper and olive oil in a culinary robot or a mixer until smooth.
> Add the red pepper sauce, olive oil and Italian seasoning. Deal Until well mixed.

131 ONION SMOTHERED STEAK

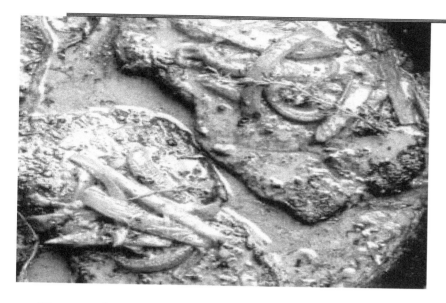

Preparation: 10 mins
Cook: 20 mins.
Serving: 8

INGREDIENTS

- ❖ ¼ cup of flour
- ❖ 1/8 TSP. pepper
- ❖ Round steak of 1 ½ lb, 3/4 "thick
- ❖ 2 tablespoons. oil
- ❖ 1 cup of water
- ❖ 1 tablespoon. the vinegar
- ❖ 1 clove garlic, mined
- ❖ 1 bay sheet
- ❖ ¼ c. Dried thyme, crushed
- ❖ 3 medium onions, sliced

INSTRUCTIONS

- ➢ Cut the steak into 8 equal portions. Combine Flour and pepper and fur in meat.
- ➢ Heat the oil in a pan and brown meat on both sides. Remove from the pan and set aside.

- Combine water, vinegar, garlic, bay sheet and thyme in the pan. Bring to a boil.
- Place the meat in this mixture and cover with Sliced onions. Cover and simmer 1 hour.

1 serving = 2 oz. Meat = 2 proteins, 1 low potassium vegetable, 1 medium potassium vegetable, 2 fat.

132 ROASTED RED PEPPER PIZZA

Preparation: 10 mins
Cook: 12 mins.
Serving: 6

INGREDIENT
- 1 refrigerated pizza paste
- 1 Grilled red flag of 7 oz, drained
- 1 clove with garlic
- 1/2 tablespoon extra-virgin olive oil
- 1/4 teaspoon salt
- 2 and 1/2 cup of mozzarella cheese shredded
- 1/2 cup of ricotta cheese
- 1/2 tablespoon Parmesan cheese
- 5-6 fresh basil leaves, chopped
- Extra virgin olive oil, garlic powder and crust salt

INSTRUCTIONS
- Preheat the oven to 425. Slightly spray a pizza stove with cooking sprayer. Open the pizza dough and roll on a floured surface until you have a circle of 12 "(see above in post for a more detailed explanation of the best way to deploy the pizza). Cook for 8 minutes Then remove from the oven.
- In a culinary robot or mixer, mix roasted red peppers, garlic clove, salt and 1/2 tablespoon oil.

> After the pizza dough is pre-cooked, cover it with mozzarella cheese, leaving a small border for the crust. If you think he needs more cheese depending on the size of your pizza dough, all means adds more cheese! Once the crust was covered with mozzarella, the spoon on the top in small shoulders with ricotta cheese, then sprinkle on the top of the parmesan cheese, then drizzle the roast red pepper sauce. With a building brush (or you can use a paper towel such as a brush) coat the crust with extra virgin olive oil and sprinkle very lightly with garlic powder and a little salt. Cook at 425 for 10-12 minutes until the crust is crispy and the cheese is slightly brown and sparkling.

> Top with chopped basil. Let cool a little, then cut and eat

133 TANGY BOX & KABOBS OF VEGETABLES

INGREDIENTS

- ❖ 3 TISP. Honey
- ❖ 3 TISP.FRESH Lime Juice
- ❖ 1 C. canola oil
- ❖ 5 TER. Ms. Dash® extra spruce or original mix
- ❖ 1 lb ox shot steak, coupe in 1 ½ "squares
- ❖ ½ big red pepper, cut in 1 "squares
- ❖ ½ big green pepper, cut in 1 "squares
- ❖ 1 medium red onion, coupe in quarters
- ❖ 1 zucchini, cut into ½ "slices

INSTRUCTIONS

> Dip the wooden skewers in water for approx. 10 minutes (to prevent them from burning during cooking) Mix honey, lime juice, oil and Ms Dash In a big bowl. Add in all remaining ingredients and Mix slightly to carefully coat the seasoning mixture.

> Wire of meat and vegetables alternately on skewers.

> Place the skewers on the grilling stove rack so that Kabobs are About 3-5 inches of heat. Grill 8-12 minutes or until Desired drawing. You can also cook on the barbecue!

Note: If you do not have skewers, the Kabob Shish the ingredients can be grills in a saucepan. Follow the steps 1 and 2 above. Sprinkle a few c. marinade On vegetables and grills until tender, stirring once.

Made 4 servings

1 serving = 3 protein, 1 medium potassium vegetable

134 ROASTED RED PEPPER SAUCE

INGREDIENTS
- ❖ 1 whole red pepper, roast
- ❖ 1-2 garlic cloves
- ❖ Dash - Black pepper
- ❖ 1 C. olive oil

INSTRUCTIONS
> Roasted pepper in the grid or barbecue until the skin becomes black.
> Leave the pepper cool and then take off the skin and throw. Mash potatoes Peppers, garlic, black pepper and olive oil in a culinary robot or mixer up smooth.

Made 1 serving

FISH & SEAFOOD

135 LINGUINE WITH GARLIC AND SHRIMP

INGREDIENTS

- ❖ 2 ½ liters water
- ❖ ¾ pounds of linguine pasta, uncooked
- ❖ 2 tablespoons. Olive oil
- ❖ 2 heads of garlic, integer
- ❖ Shrimp ½ book, peeled and cleaned
- ❖ 1 cup of flat parsley
- ❖ 1 tablespoon. Lemon juice
- ❖ Black pepper to taste

INSTRUCTIONS

- ➢ Boil water in a large pot. Add pasta and cook for 10 minutes or until tender.
- ➢ 2. While the pasta burned, garlic cloves separate, leaving the skin. Heat pods in a medium heat stove, stirring often. Garlic is ready when it darkens and becomes soft to touch. The skin will be easy to remove. Remove the garlic from the pan and take off the skin.
- ➢ 3. Heat the olive oil into the pan and return to the garlic peeled in the casserole. Cook the garlic to Golden. (Cloves can be cut in two or left whole).
- ➢ 4. Add parsley and shrimp and cook 1 to 2 minutes until Shrimps become pink.
- ➢ 5. Drain pasta and reserve 1 cup of liquid. Add pasta Poor with shrimp and garlic. Mix all ingredients together and add the cup of reserved liquid.
- ➢ 6. Add lemon juice, black pepper, mix and serve.

Made 4 servings. 1 serving = 2 cup = 1½ meat, 4 starch, 1 low potassium vegetable

NOTE

Adjust the shrimp part for a higher or lower protein diet. For a lower carbohydrate power, divide the recipe into 6 portions instead of 4 servings. Carbohydrates are reduced to 44 g, 3 choices of carbohydrates.

136 SALMON STUFFED PASTA SHELLS

INGREDIENTS
- ❖ 24 Jumbo pasta shells
- ❖ 2 eggs, beaten
- ❖ 2 cups of creamy cottage cheese
- ❖ (regular or without salt)
- ❖ ¼ cup of chopped onion
- ❖ 1 red or green pepper, in cubes
- ❖ 2 teaspoons. Dry parsley
- ❖ ½ teaspoon Finely grated lemon peel
- ❖ 1 can salmon; Rinse, drained
- ❖ and scales
- ❖ 1 cup of rich coffee

Dill sauce
- ❖ 1 ½ teaspoon. margarine
- ❖ 1 ½ teaspoon. flour
- ❖ 1/8 teaspoon. Pepper
- ❖ 1 tablespoon. lemon juice
- ❖ 1 ½ cup of rich coffee
- ❖ 2 teaspoons. Dill leaves

INSTRUCTIONS
- ➢ Cook pasta according to the instructions of the package; drain; cool on waxed paper or aluminum leaf to avoid paste.
- ➢ Combine eggs, cottage cheese, onion, pepper, Parsley, lemon zest and salmon.
- ➢ Pour the Rich coffee into a 9 "x 2" cooking dish slightly oiled.

- ➤ Fill each pasta shell with filling. Organize Shells in the baking dish; Cover with aluminum foil. Cook at 350 ° F For 30 to 35 minutes, or until hot and sparkling.
- ➤ While shells make cooking, fondue margarine in a small pan on Medium cooking temperature. Stir in flour and pepper. Remove heat; Gradually add the coffee launder or rice drink, stirring until smooth. Return to medium heat; boil constantly. Reduce heat and simmer for 1 minute. Remove heat and stir from dill juice and lemon.
- ➤ Remove the oven dishes. Organize shells on a tray, Serve with dill sauce.

6 servings, 1 serving = 4 shell = 2 choice of protein and 2 starches.

Water sauce

137 BAKED TILAPIA FISH WITH GARLIC SAUCE

Preparation: 10 mins
Cook time: 15 mins.
Serving: 2

INGREDIENTS
- ❖ 500 grimy tilapia fillets (3-4 steaks)
- ❖ 2 sliced thick medium onions
- ❖ 2 cups of peppers sliced thick middle strips
- ❖ ¼ cup of sinful molten butter
- ❖ 1 tablespoon of chopped garlic
- ❖ 1 tablespoon of fresh lemon juice
- ❖ 2 teaspoons of Italian seasoning (or mixed dry grass)
- ❖ 1 teaspoon of red chili flakes (taste for taste)
- ❖ Salt and pepper according to taste
- ❖ 3-4 slice of fresh lemon

INSTRUCTIONS

- ➢ For mixing marinade, melted butter, garlic, lemon juice, herbs, chili flakes, salt and pepper in a bowl.
- ➢ In a baking tray, add the onion and sliced pepper. Add a couple of spoons from the previous marinade. Mix well.
- ➢ Then place the tilapia fillets. Brush the rest of the marinated uniformly on both sides.
- ➢ Place the slice of lemon.
- ➢ Bake in a preheated oven at 200 c / 400 F for 12-15 minutes.
- ➢ Serve in a bed of rice along with vegetables. Saving spoon of lemon butter from the pan.

NUTRITION

Serving: 100g | Calories: 528kcal | Carbohydrates: 19g | Protein: 53g | Gordo: 27g | Hat: 16g | Cholesterol: 186mg | Sodium: 151mg | Potassium: 1176mg | Fiber: 5g | Sugar: 8g | Vitamin A: 1410iu | Vitamin C: 132.1mg | Calcium: 95mg | Iron: 2.5mg.

PORK

138 CRANBERRY SPRERIBS

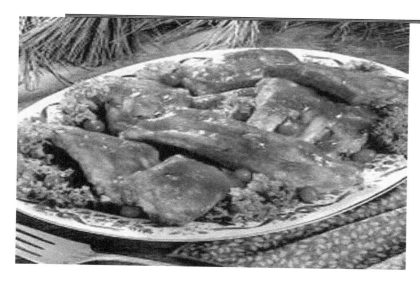

Preparation: 35 mins
Cook time: 1Hrs.
Serving: 6

INGREDIENTS
- ❖ Spareribs of 4 pounds
- ❖ 1 box (14 ounces) whole cranberry sauce
- ❖ 1 box (10 ounces) beef sauce
- ❖ 1/2 cup of orange marmalade
- ❖ 1/4 cup of lemon juice
- ❖ 1/8 ground cinnamon coffee spoon
- ❖ 1 teaspoon of vinegar

INSTRUCTIONS
- ➢ Cut ribs into server pieces; Place in a Dutch oven or a large kettle. Cover with water; bring to a boil. Lower the temperature; Cover and simmer for 45 minutes.

> Meanwhile, in an average saucepan, combine cranberry sauce, sauce, marmalade, lemon juice and cinnamon; bring to a boil. Lower the temperature; Simmer for 10-15 minutes or thickened, stirring occasionally. Remove heat; Stir in vinegar. Empty the coast; Place with meat up in a 13 "greased. x 9-in. Flat cooking. Pour 2-1 / 2 cups of sauce on ribs. Cover and cook at 400 ° for 20 minutes. Discover and cook 15-20 minutes more or until the meat is tender, disengage every 5 minutes with a remaining sauce.

NUTRITIONAL
1 each: 755 calories, 43 g of fat (saturated grease of 16g), 173 mg of cholesterol, 460 mg sodium, 100 g of carbohydrates (36g sugars, 1g fibers), 42g protein.

139 HERB-RUBBED PORK TENDERLOIN

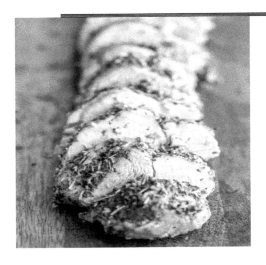

Preparation: 10 mins
Cook time: 35 mins.
Serving: 4

INGREDIENTS
- ❖ 2 cloves garlic
- ❖ 1 teaspoon dried basil
- ❖ 1 C. Thyme
- ❖ 1 C. Dried rosemary tea

- ❖ Freshly cracked black pepper
- ❖ 1/2 c.
- ❖ 2 tablespoons of olive oil
- ❖ 1,33 lb pork net

INSTRUCTIONS

- ➤ Preheat the oven to 400°F. Chop garlic. Add the dried basil, thyme and rosemary to a small dish. Use your hands to slightly crush the dried rosemary. Add garlic, olive oil, salt and a small black pepper freshly cracked to bowl and move to combine.
- ➤ Place the pork net on a pastry plate or a cooking dish. Rub the oil and grass mixture over the entire pork surface, including below.
- ➤ Place the cooktop in the preheated oven and roasting pork for about 35 minutes, or until the internal temperature reads at least 145 ° F. Leave the pig to rest at room temperature for 10 minutes before to decide and serve.

NUTRITION

Service: 1serving · Calories: 280.1Kcal · Carbohydrates: 2.1g · Protein: 28.6g · Fat: 17.53g · Sodium: 828.3mg · Fiber: 0.3g

140 ITALIAN PORK CUTLETS

Preparation: 10 mins
Cook time: 25 mins.
Serving: 4

INGREDIENTS

- ❖ 4 boneless pork chops (4 ounces)

- ❖ Sea salt
- ❖ Freshly ground pepper
- ❖ 1 cup of flour
- ❖ 3 big eggs
- ❖ 1 cup of Italian style bread crumbs
- ❖ 1 teaspoon of dried parsley
- ❖ 1 teaspoon of dried thyme
- ❖ Olive oil

DIRECTION

- ➢ Take your boneless pork chops and drive them a slim place individually on a work board and cover with wax paper or a clear envelope. Take your mallet and marcez skinny.
- ➢ Season both sides slightly with salt and pepper.
- ➢ Get out 3 large bowls or plates. Add the flour into one then whip the eggs in one, then the crumbs of bread. For bread chips, add it to parsley and thyme and combine well. Align a mounting string.
- ➢ Heat a large saucepan with enough olive oil to cover the bottom. Let it heat very hot on average temperature.
- ➢ Dip the chopper in the flour then the egg and finally the crumbs of bread. Add the chop to the hot prohibition and cook every side for about 3 minutes. If you make lots on a plate and cover with aluminum foil.
- ➢ Serve with a salad and / or your favorite vegetables. Sprinkle with extra-virgin olive oil and a corner of lemon.

141 PEPPERCORN PORK CHOPS

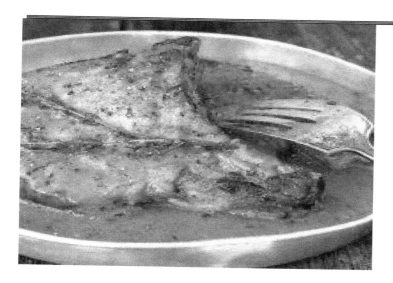

Preparation: 15 mins
Cook time: 20 mins.
Serving: 2

INGREDIENTS

- ❖ 2 pork chops cut from a two-inch thick bone, blocked if you like * See notes
- ❖ 1 1/2 c. Butter
- ❖ 1 tablespoon of olive oil
- ❖ Salt pepper and freshly ground
- ❖ 2 tablespoons of flour
- ❖ Sauce:
- ❖ 1 tablespoon of butter
- ❖ 1/4 cup of ulphits very finely chopped or onion
- ❖ 2 - 3 teaspoons of crushed pepper, black, green or red or a mixture
- ❖ 1/4 - 1/3 cup of red or white wine or Marsala dry wine
- ❖ 1 cup of chicken bouillon or beef
- ❖ 1/2 c. Dijon mustard, optional
- ❖ 2 - 3 thyme twigs

- 1/4 cup of thick cream, or lighter cream and add more thickener
- Salt and freshly ground pepper, to taste
- Thicken the sauce (add only as necessary):
- 2 CMSP corn corn
- 1 tablespoon of water

INSTRUCTIONS

- Preheat the oven to 400F.
- Heat olive oil and butter in a stove with the oven or cast iron on medium-high heat. Park dry pork chops and season with salt and pepper. The dispersion flour on the plate and the dredge pork chops slightly on both sides. Sear chops in a hot stove until it is slightly golden on both sides. Pop the pan with preheated oven pork chops and cook until the pork reaches 135f, about 10-12 minutes (depending on the thickness of the chops). Note that it's a bit undercut because he will cook a little further on the stove and a little more than that is resting, he will arrive at the 145F recommended at the end.
- Remove from the oven and place over the middle-edge on the stove. Quickly remove the chops on the stove, then remove it into a plate to rest.
- At the hot stove, add 1 tablespoon of butter, onions and peppers and stir until the onions are golden, about 1 minute. Add wine and cook, agitation until especially evaporated, about 1 minute. Add a broth, dijon mustard and thyme sprigs. Reduce the heat to medium and let the sauce simmer / reduce for a few minutes. Add cream, then salt and pepper to taste. Thicken the sauce, mix cornstarch and water in a small bowl, stirring to smooth. Add a little bit to your hot sauce, stirring until the desired thickness is reached.
- Spoon to hot sauce on pork chops. Complete a generous grind of freshly ground pepper.

NUTRITION

Calories: 578kcal, Carbohydrates: 16g, Protein: 51g, FAT: 41g, Saturated grease: 19g, Cholesterol: 234 mg, Sodium: 717mg, Potassium: 962mg, Vitamin A: 950iu, Vitamin C: 10.6 mg, Calcium: 73 mg, Iron: 2.4 mg.

142 HONEY GARLIC PORK CHOPS RECIPE

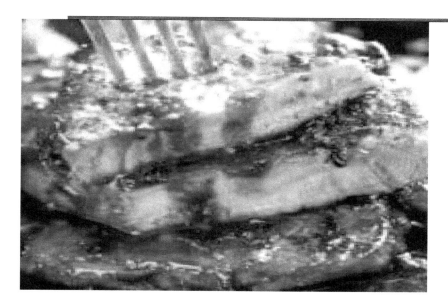

Preparation: 10 mins
Cook time: 12 mins.
Serving: 4

INGREDIENT

- ❖ 4 pork entrance or out
- ❖ Salt and pepper, until season
- ❖ 1 teaspoon of garlic powder
- ❖ 2 tablespoons of olive oil
- ❖ 1 tablespoon of unsalted butter
- ❖ 6 cloves of garlic, chopped
- ❖ 1/4 cup dear

- ❖ 1/4 cup of water (or chicken broth)
- ❖ 2 tablespoons of rice vinegar rice (or apple cider vinegar, or white vinegar)

INSTRUCTIONS

- ➢ Heating broiler ovens (or grill) on medium heat. The meat season with salt, pepper and garlic powder before being cooked.
- ➢ Heat the oil in a skillet or a pan over medium heat until it's hot. Chopped Sear on both sides to golden and cooked (about 4-5 minutes each side). Transfer to the plate; Set aside.
- ➢ Reduce heat to the media. Melt butter in the same skillet, scratch brownish bits from the bottom of the pan. Sauté garlic until fragrant (about 30 seconds). Add honey, water and vinegar. It adds hot to medium and keeps cooking until the sauce is reduced and thickens a little (about 3-4 minutes), while stirring occasionally.
- ➢ Add pigs back into the skillet, baste generously with sauce and grilled / grill for 1-2 minutes, or until the end is a little charred.
- ➢ Decorate with parsley and serve vegetables, rice, pasta or with salads.

NUTRITION

Calories: 332kcal | Carbohydrates: 15g | Protein: 29g | FAT: 12G | Saturated grease: 5G | Cholesterol: 104mg | Sodium: 68mg | Potassium: 337mg | Sugar: 14g | Vitamin A: 175iu | Vitamin C: 1.4mg | Calcium: 18mg | Iron: 0.8 mg

POULTRY

143 BASIL CHICKEN

INGREDIENTS
- ❖ 4 halves of skinless chicken breast (cutting visible grease)
- ❖ 1/3 cup of margarine, fondue
- ❖ ¼ cup of fresh basil, minced or 2 c. dried basil
- ❖ 1 tablespoon. Parmesan, grated cheese
- ❖ ¼ c. garlic powder
- ❖ ¼ c. Ms. Dash SEL-Fersonation Duration
- ❖ Fresh Basil Sprigs, Optional Garnish

INSTRUCTIONS
- ➤ Preheat the oven to 325 ° F. Place the halves of chicken breast In a glass pan.
- ➤ Drill each chest with a fork several times to allow mix for the season and flavor as he cooking.
- ➤ Melt Margarine in a bowl of glass mixture in the microwave.
- ➤ Start at 15 seconds and stir to distribute heat.
- ➤ To melt margarine, add the basil, Parmesan cheese,
- ➤ AIL and MRS.DASH® powder.
- ➤ Stir mixture with a fork or whip.
- ➤ Pour the mixture evenly on the chicken breasts making sure that Parmesan cheese is distributed smoothly.

> Cook at discovery, giving every 10 minutes with mixture of the pan, for a total of about 25 minutes or until the juice in the chicken is clear, not pink.

Made 4 servings

1 servant = 3 proteins

144 BARBECUE LEMON CHICKEN

INGREDIENTS
- ❖ 4 boneless chicken breasts
- ❖ 1 lemon juice
- ❖ 2 tsp. olive oil
- ❖ 1 garlic clove, minced
- ❖ ½ tsp. dried overall
- ❖ Cayenne pepper pinch

INSTRUCTIONS
> Remove the skin from the chicken. In a shallow dish, arrange

> Chicken in one layer.

> In a small dish, combine lemon juice, oil, garlic, oregano and Cayenne; mix well. Pour on the chicken and turn to handle on both sides. Let stand at room temperature for 20 minutes or cover and refrigerate up to 6 hours.

> On grilled grill or grill pan, cook the chicken for 4-5 minutes on each side or until the meat is no longer pink inside.

Made 4 servings, 1 servant = 3 proteins

145 CHICKEN CURRY RECIPE

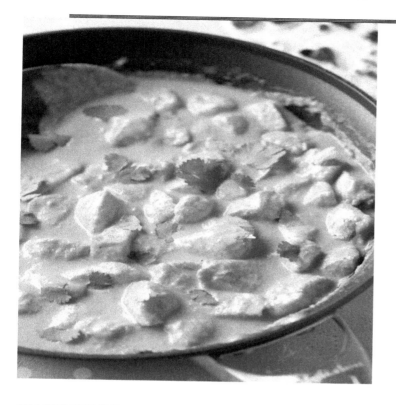

INGREDIENTS

- ❖ 1 lb (450 g) chicken, no skin
- ❖ 1 clove of garlic, crushed or garlic to taste
- ❖ 1 medium onion, chopped
- ❖ Small amount of canola or vegetable oil
- ❖ the water
- ❖ ¼ c. pepper
- ❖ 1 tablespoon. curry powder
- ❖ 1 C. cornstarch
- ❖ 1 oz. (25 g) Margarine low salty non hydrogenate

INSTRUCTIONS

- ➢ Cut the chicken. Fry the onion and garlic to brown.
- ➢ Add chicken and make a fry gently in small amount of oil.

- ➤ In a separate saucepan, mix margarine and whip in cornstarch.

- ➤ Add some water while doing this to form a dough.

- ➤ Add in water (up to 1 cup) and whisk Curry powder and pepper.

- ➤ Add a chicken sauce and boil to thicken and reduce the sauce.

- ➤ Reduce heat, cover and simmer until cooking.

- ➤ Add more water if necessary, to avoid engraving.

Made 4 servings

1 servant = 3 proteins

This dish is delicious with rice or boiled pasta! Enjoy!

146 CHICKEN FINGERS

INGREDIENTS
- ❖ Breast cup
- ❖ 2 tablespoons. Parmesan cheese
- ❖ ¼ c. pepper
- ❖ 1 ½ tsp. dried thyme
- ❖ ¾ tsp. Each garlic and onion powder
- ❖ 4 chicken breast (halves), boneless, skinless
- ❖ (Cut in 1 "bands)
- ❖ ¼ mug of non-hydrogenated margarine, fondue

INSTRUCTIONS
- ➤ Preheat the oven to 400 ° F. Combine the first 5 ingredients. Soak
- ➤ chicken in molten margarine; Then coat with mixture

- ➢ Ingredients. Place a slightly greased rack on a cookie sheet.
- ➢ Cook 10 minutes, turn and cook for 10 minutes more.
- ➢ Gives 12 chicken fingers.

1 chicken finger = 1 protein, ½ starch

147 CHICKEN SATAYS

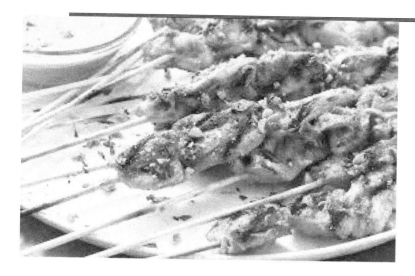

INGREDIENTS
- ❖ 4 chicken breasts (about 1 lb / 500g)
- ❖ 2 tablespoons. olive oil
- ❖ 2 tablespoons. Red wine vinegar
- ❖ 1 tablespoon. McCormick No table Added Salt Shake seasoning®
- ❖ 24 bamboo skewers

INSTRUCTIONS
- ➢ Cut the chicken into 24 thin bands, ½ "(1 cm) wide. Medium bowl or self-seal plastic bag, mix the oil, vinegar and McCormick No salt added the seasoning table. Add Chicken straps and mix to coat. Cover and refrigerate At least 30 min., or night, turning from time to time.

> ➤ During this time, soak bamboo skewers in the water for 30 minutes, Eliminate the chicken from the marinade and the thread on each skewer. Grill or grill about 5 min. by side or until not Longer pink. Discard any remaining marinade.

Gives 12 servings

1 serving = 2 satrapy, = 1 portion of proteins

SAUCES & SALAD DRESSINGS

148 BARBEQUE SAUCE

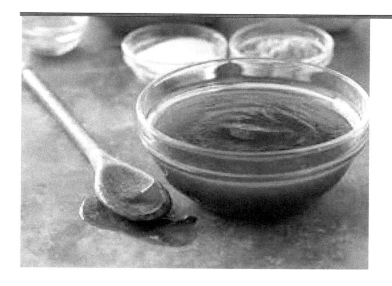

INGREDIENTS

- ❖ 1/3 cup of corn oil
- ❖ ½ cup of tomato juice
- ❖ 1 tablespoon brown sugar
- ❖ 1 garlic clove
- ❖ 1 tablespoon. paprika
- ❖ ¼ cup of vinegar
- ❖ 1 C. pepper
- ❖ 1/3 cup of water
- ❖ ¼ c. onion powder

INSTRUCTIONS

- ➢ Combine all the ingredients. Simmer

> - for about 20 minutes.
> - Refrigerate unused portions in a closed container.
> - Made 8 servings. 1 serving = 2 c.

For those on a low potassium regime, 2 tablespoons. = ½ medium potassium vegetable.

149 BASIC DRESSING

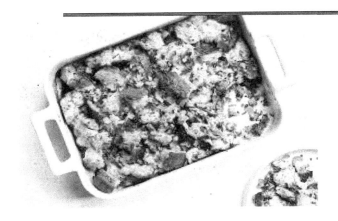

INGREDIENTS
- ❖ ¼ cup of red wine vinegar
- ❖ ¼ c. garlic powder
- ❖ ¼ c. dried mustard
- ❖ ½ tsp. sugar
- ❖ ¼ cup of water
- ❖ ¼ c. ground black pepper
- ❖ 2 tablespoons. Fresh lemon juice
- ❖ 1 cup of corn or olive oil
- ❖ (Made 1-1 ½ cups)

INSTRUCTIONS

Combine all the ingredients and pour into a container with a

Cover well adapted and shake. Shop, cover in the refrigerator.

150 CURRY DRESSING

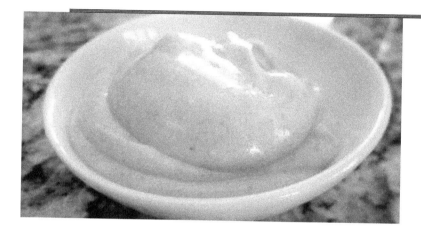

INGREDIENTS

- ❖ 1 C. curry powder
- ❖ 1/8 TSP. grounded ginger
- ❖ ½ cup of basic vinaigrette *
- ❖ Mix well. Shop, cover in the refrigerator.

151 ITALIAN DRESSING

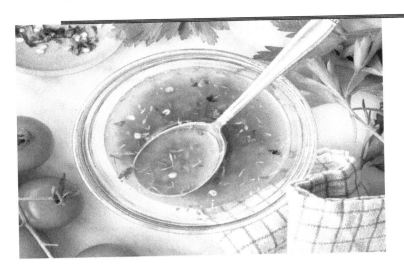

INGREDIENTS
- ❖ 2 tsp. Dried overall
- ❖ 1 C. dried basil
- ❖ 1 C. dried tractions
- ❖ ½ tsp. sugar
- ❖ ½ cup of basic vinaigrette

INSTRUCTIONS
- ➢ Mix well.
- ➢ Shop, cover in the refrigerator.
- ➢ Can use these dressings as a marinade for fish, poultry and meat

152 CREAMY VINAIGRETTE DRESSING

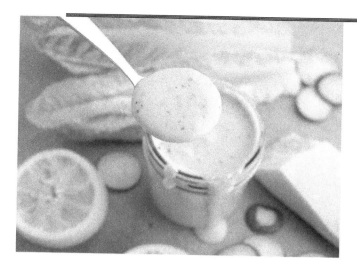

INGREDIENTS

- ❖ 2 tablespoons. cider vinegar
- ❖ 2 tablespoons. Lime or lemon juice
- ❖ 1 clove with garlic, minced
- ❖ 1 C. Dijon's mustard
- ❖ 1 C. cumin powder
- ❖ ½ cup of sour cream
- ❖ 2 tablespoons. olive oil
- ❖ ¼ c. black pepper

INSTRUCTIONS

- ➢ Combine all the ingredients and mix well.
- ➢ Pour into the salad balloon. Coldness.

153 HONEY DRESSING

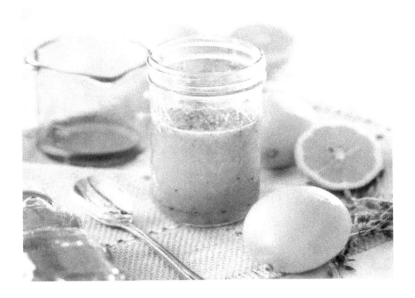

INGREDIENTS

- ½ cup) sugar
- 1 C. dried mustard
- 1 C. paprika
- ½ cup of honey
- ¼ cup of vinegar
- 2 tablespoons. lemon juice
- 1 C. grated onion
- 1 cup of salad oil

INSTRUCTIONS

- Mix dry ingredients - add honey, vinegar, lemon juice
- and onion.
- Beat with mixer; Slowly add oil, beating constantly.
- Ideal for vegetable or fruit salads!

- ➢ Marinades
- ➢ Use one or the other to marinate 1 lb of poultry, beef or pork at 1 lb.

154 TERRIYAKI MARINADE

INGREDIENTS

- ❖ 2 tablespoons. Salt soy sauce
- ❖ 2 tablespoons. Baking sherry or apple juice
- ❖ 1 C. dried ginger
- ❖ 2 tablespoons. canola oil
- ❖ 1 C. brown sugar
- ❖ 1 clove garlic, mined
- ❖ ½ tsp. pepper

155 HERB MARINADE

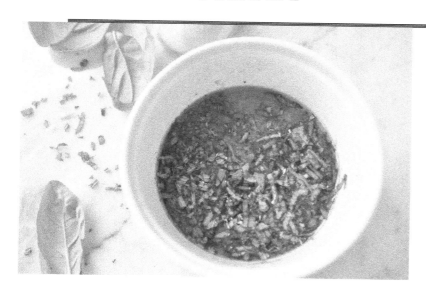

INGREDIENTS

- ❖ ½ Cup of lemon juice
- ❖ 1 c. Honey
- ❖ 1/3 cup of cooking oil or olive oil
- ❖ 1 garlic clove, finely chopped
- ❖ 1 tablespoon. Chopped fresh parsley
- ❖ 1 c. Dried basil
- ❖ ¼ c. dried overall

INSTRUCTIONS

- ➢ Combine ingredients and mix well. Place poultry, beef or Pork in a sealing plastic bag. Pour the marinade into the bag and refrigerate 4 to 24 hours. Remove the meat and throw the marinade. Cook meat as directed.
- ➢ For those of a low potassium diet, count the herbal marinade as ½ fruit serving

156 APPLE JUICE MARINADE

INGREDIENTS

- ❖ ½ cup of apple juice
- ❖ ¼ cup of low salt soy sauce
- ❖ ¼ cup of honey
- ❖ 2 tablespoons. lemon juice
- ❖ ½ tsp. garlic powder
- ❖ ¼ c. dried mustard
- ❖ ¼ c. grounded ginger

INSTRUCTIONS

- Combine ingredients and mix well. Place 1 LB boned or 1 ½ lbs poultry bone or pork in a sealing plastic bag.
- Pour the marinade into the bag and refrigerate 4 to 24 hours.
- Remove the meat from the bag and throw the marinade.
- Cook meat as directed.
- For poor potassium regimes, count above 1 fruit service.

157 OIL AND VINEGAR

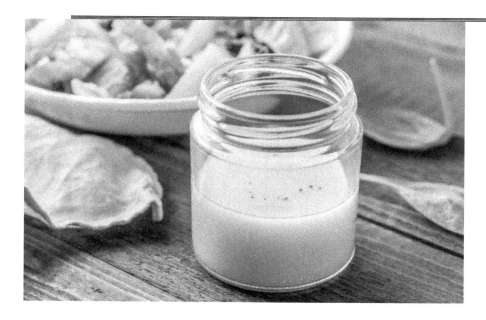

INGREDIENTS
- ¼ cup of balsamic vinegar
- ¼ cup of olive oil
- ¼ c. paprika
- ¼ c. grated Parmesan cheese
- Pepper pinch

INSTRUCTIONS
- Whip all the ingredients.

> Mix with a salad.

158 PICKLED PINEAPPLE

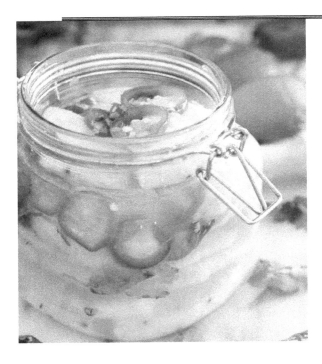

INGREDIENTS

- ❖ 3 cans (15 oz.) Pineapple pieces
- ❖ 1 cup of sugar (or Splenda)
- ❖ 8 pods (integer)
- ❖ Cup of vinegar
- ❖ A 4 "cinnamon stick

INSTRUCTIONS

- ➢ Drain the pineapple. Save the cup juices.
- ➢ Combine backed up pineapple juice with rest Ingredients and heat 10 minutes.
- ➢ Add pineapple and bring to a boil.
- ➢ Remove from heat and put in pots.

> Store in the refrigerator Try this to add a pizza to your meat or chicken!

1 serving = 2-4 c. = ½ dessert of fruits.

159 BASIC SEASONING

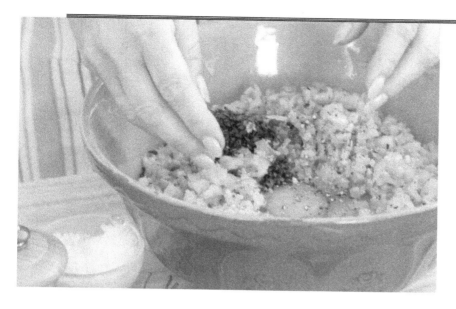

INGREDIENTS

- ❖ 2 tablespoons. paprika
- ❖ 1 tablespoon. dried mustard
- ❖ 1 tablespoon. garlic powder
- ❖ 1 tablespoon. onion powder
- ❖ 1 C. pepper
- ❖ 1 C. thyme
- ❖ 1 C. basil

160 CHINESE SEASONING

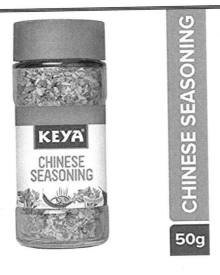

INGREDIENTS

- ❖ 4 tsp. grounded ginger
- ❖ 2 tablespoons. onion powder
- ❖ 1 tablespoon. The seeds of crushed anise
- ❖ 2 tsp. Land allspice
- ❖ ½ tsp. ground clove
- ❖ 2 tsp. Sesame seeds

161 ITALIAN SEASONING

INGREDIENTS

- ❖ 2 tablespoons. garlic powder
- ❖ 1 tablespoon. parsley
- ❖ 1 tablespoon. basil

- ❖ 1 tablespoon. Oregano
- ❖ ½ tsp. pepper
- ❖ ½ tsp. thyme
- ❖ 2 tsp. onion powder
- ❖ Is about ½ cup. Mix the ingredients together and store in an airtight container.

162 SEASONING TACO

INGREDIENTS

- ❖ 3 c. onion powder
- ❖ 2 tablespoons. cumin powder
- ❖ 1 ½ tsp. chili powder
- ❖ ½ tsp. Cayenne
- ❖ 1 C. garlic powder
- ❖ Is about ½ cup. Mix the ingredients together and store
- ❖ in an airtight container.
- ❖

CPSIA information can be obtained
at www.ICGtesting.com
Printed in the USA
LVHW060000260521
688447LV00017B/827